A Complete Low Carb Lifestyle

An Executive Chefs Low Carb Lifestyle Culinary Guide

By

Gregory Pryor C.E.C.

ISBN: 1-4107-9400-8 (e-book)
ISBN: 1-4107-9399-0 (Paperback)
ISBN: 1-4107-9398-2 (Dust Jacket)

Library of Congress Control Number: 2003096306

This book is printed on acid free paper.

Printed in the United States of America
Bloomington, IN

1stBooks – rev. 09/24/03

CONTENTS

Dedicated to the memory of
Robert C. Atkins M.D. 1930-2003

Whose memories shall live on, in the lives of all the people he has touched, and whose lives will forever be changed, by his determination to rid the world of obesity and its associated health issues.

Gregory Pryor

ACKNOWLEDGMENTS

I wish to take this moment to acknowledge the many people to whom I am grateful for the support and motivation given me to finally taking the step to writing this book. I feel I must first pay special tribute to Dr. Robert Atkins and his wonderful wife Veronica for the many efforts and tireless years of devotion Dr. Atkins, with the support of his wife, have given to such a worthy cause. Despite all the years of negative encounters, we would not be shaping our lives towards a low carb lifestyle were it not for his unwavering dedication and brilliance. I would also like to express my sincere appreciation for the opportunity to have worked with Dr. Atkins and the wonderful members of the Atkins Group and staff.

I wish to also share my deepest heart felt thanks to my wife Susan, for understanding the passion this lifestyle has evolved into. Her continued praise and motivation to follow my dreams have and always are the unwavering support needed to accomplish my goals and dreams.

I wish also to thank all of my family members, Cindy, Chrissy and Gregory for being supportive of their father at times when many thought I had lost my marbles. To my Mother for also believing her only son was not just being a fanatic about this lifestyle and to my Sister Terri for being my biggest fan and test subject for many recipes. (Even though she does not like to cook). To my wife's parents Robert and Margaret for their continued moral support at times when I was nearly being anti-social during the many times I was researching and creating recipes.

Thank you to Steven Weege for the hours spent finding my missed periods, commas and redundant words that I missed on countless times reading my own writing.

Most importantly to the entire Low Carb enthusiast that have made the decision to take control of your lives. But especially to those that have taken this time to read my book.

God Bless you all.

INTRODUCTION

This is not just a cookbook. Nor is it simply a collection of recipes low in carbohydrates. What this book is, however, is a collection of knowledge, inspirations, guidance, and moral support that will be your key to a successful Low Carb Lifestyle. Contained within these pages is an exploration of the myths and facts associated with Low Carb Lifestyle, and the dos and don'ts for success. Because of the continued success and interest in the Low Carb Lifestyle, many culinary myths exist both in print and in idea. My purpose for writing this book is to share with you the knowledge and understanding of food, culinary use of and the classic applications of cooking rich, flavorful, satisfying, rewarding meals that are the key to a satisfying Low Carb Lifestyle.

In today's fast paced lifestyle, exist many reasons people may choose to ignore the Low Carb Lifestyle, as a way to both control their weight and improve their overall health. Many arguments exist about what correct diet serves our lifestyle best. One fact for certain (in my humble opinion) is that the word diet is the first strike in the batting order. What we will be exploring in these pages is a Lifestyle, **not a diet**. The decision to control our weight is one that takes a strong commitment, but also, as with any change we make in our lifestyles, change never comes easy.

My goal is to support and motivate those who have made a commitment to themselves and their loved ones to take back control of their lifestyle. As we can agree, the benefits of proper weight management may be the most important action that we can take control of ourselves. Today, more than ever before, weight control is the greater issue. My personal beliefs and experiences have proven to me that the simplest and easiest of all weight control changes we can make in our life is the control of carbohydrate intake in our daily diet.

CLASSICAL AND SENSIBLE

What we are going to explore further in this book is both the classic and sensible approach to Low Carb Cuisine. First the classic approach. Classical cuisine-by-design historically was, and still is a Low Carb cuisine. Here we will take the Classical Cuisine design, and incorporate into our daily life styles. Let's look at Classical Cuisine; it consists of rich beef, chicken, fish and pork dishes. With classically flavorful rich beef and veal stock, butter sauces, beef and wine sauces, and other rich and robust flavored cream sauces. Also we will look at the wonderful use of *"reductions"*. We will examine the use of Chicken Stocks, Fish Stocks and Veal Stocks to create those rich flavorful Sauces, such as Demi-Glace, Volute and Fumet's.

By taking Classical Cuisine and adjusting the ingredients and techniques we can incorporate this into our daily lifestyle. Many of the techniques, flavors and ingredients from this classical era are still widely used today. In today's search for Low Carb recipes and menus one only has to look to the internet or any major bookstore shelf to recognize the demand for satisfying and flavorful yet (not so boring recipes). Many of these recipes that we find now on the internet and in Low Carb cookbooks overlook the obvious. The obvious being the Low Carb Classical Cuisine.

When I look at many of these recipes, and yes I have tried many of them, most I have found miss the mark. Our goal is to get back on track, find that mark and simplify our Low Carb Lifestyle. What we will not do in this book is try to recreate the wheel. What I mean by that is we are going to work with basic common available ingredients and products to create succulent satisfying nutritious recipes and menus. My biggest complaint about many of the internet recipes, and even some of those in print, is the constant attempt to reinvent the wheel, in this case, classical recipes. Let's look at a few. With the introduction of Splenda®, we can now make basic ice-cream with minimal carbs. Let's look at some of the sauces. Butter sauces, rich veal stock reductions, mayonnaise and cream sauces are all low in carbs in their classic preparation.

With the increase in demand for Low Carb products, technology and science are starting to recognize, the thirty to fifty million Americans that have chosen a Low Carb Lifestyle. A perfect example is the introduction of Splenda®, a sugar substitute. I am certain of one thing. Once the makers of food items such as bread, pasta and other flour based products recognize that this demand equals profits, these items will soon be on our shelves as well. Now let's talk about the sensible part for a minute.

One of the toughest aspects of the Low Carb cuisine and lifestyle is accepting that many of those high carbohydrate foods that many of us feel we can't ever do without, just do not fit into this new lifestyle. Yes I know there are recipes and products out there today, especially with the advent of the internet. Breads, pastas, pancake mixes, waffle mixes, and countless other products are advertised everywhere and, in truth, some of them aren't too bad. Some however are just flat-out terrible. So what is the answer? Well from my view it is this. First and foremost, from my own experience and sharing the experience of others, the use of many of these products only further increases our cravings for such. Let me explain. Let's take bread for example. I cannot tell you the number of times that I have met people that felt that they could not live without bread. So they substituted these Low Carb mixes and products, only to be sorely disappointed, further increasing that craving. Now let's be sensible why, do you suppose that is. Let's explore this for a minute. First and foremost don't think that I do not understand the fact that many of the high carb foods appeal to so many people. If we look a little deeper, it is simple to understand. The body has learned over the years to love Carbs, to the point of creating cravings for them. As much as I would like to assure every one of you that we can create exact Low Carb replacements for many of the high carb foods, the truth is we cannot, at least not yet. Let's look at the two most commonly requested examples. And yes, the ones we miss the most; Pasta and Bread. As of the time of writing this book the science involved to create Low Carb wheat flour is not in place. Now as a result many substitute recipes and products have evolved as replacements for these two most popular High Carb products. But here is my experience with these products. Usually, most of the people I have met and talked to, or have supervised in Low Carb cuisine all share the same conclusion. These products, although similar in looks and often texture, don't satisfy that urge or craving for the actual product. Now what happens next is that craving increases and is less manageable than if we simply do without these products, till such time we have our weight under control and can enjoy (in moderation) the true products: pasta bread and even rice.

Following a Low Carb Lifestyle does not mean that we are condemned to a lifetime of never eating any of these foods. However, it does mean that until we have our weight under control, correct our metabolism and learn to be responsible about carbohydrates we have to ignore many of these items. Respectfully, once you have reached your normal weight and body mass, many of you will be able to tolerate as many as 70 grams or more of carbohydrates daily. Taking that into mind you can see that if, we plan our meals responsibly we can include those missed foods. Simply put, we either learn to train ourselves to overcome these cravings or sadly give into them. Trying these substitutions only increases our craving for the real products that we miss. So being sensible my philosophy is this, until science and technology create true Low Carb starch based products my advice is do with out. I have heard several clichés and statements over the years but none stick closer to my mind but this *"nothing tastes as good as thin feels"* So now every time you look at that loaf of bread or that bowl of pasta and all the other starch-laden foods remember that quote.

So what is the answer to all this? The answer is simple; we have to make a commitment to ourselves. We have to take control, and we have to be strong. From the recipes, suggestions, ideas and techniques that I will share with you throughout this book, it is my most sincere wish and desire that you too will come to understand the benefits of a Low Carb Lifestyle. From the recipes in this book you will see that my goal is to be practicable, sensible and, above all, create decadent meals with the most readily available items. About Bread and Pasta. In keeping with the intent of this book, I simply cannot provide you with recipes for bread and pasta using common ingredients. If you must have these Low Carb replicas I suggest you buy them. In most homes few if any of you in the past took the time and effort to make fresh bread or pasta, so why deviate from that routine? Therefore I will provide you with a few resources to buy these items if you simply cannot live without them.

WHAT'S OUR GOAL?

Assuming of course you have made a decision to control your carbohydrates, then it is my goal to share with you the advice, wisdom, techniques and choices that will be the key to your success. First let's talk about the one thing most Americans feel they can't do without, sweets and deserts. With today's many sugar substitutes there are a wide variety of sweets and desert items that I will provide recipes for later in this book. My goal is to make these available to you, low in carbs to help you to stay away from the *"real stuff"* and stick to your commitment to a Low Carb Lifestyle. Although many sugar substitutes exist (Equal, SweetnLow, Sorbitole, Mannitol and Dextrose) just to name a few, most all of these represent some form of health concern and or digestive issues. Not to mention, few (if any) provide the true characteristics of sugar when used in baking or high heat applications.

Fortunately the FDA approved the use of Splenda® in 2000. So far this has proven to be the most sugar like substitute available today. Therefore you will find all of my recipes throughout this book will contain Splenda® for any sweeteners. While most of you know this, but for the few that may not, the one thing we will not worry about is counting calories. As you will see with most of these recipes and suggestions these are designed to be Low Carb, not low calorie. Most of these recipes make a liberal use of cream, butter, cream cheese, eggs, olive oil, and occasionally nuts to create the texture and the volume of flour that we will use sparingly or not at all.

Since fats and proteins are the vast majority of calories consumed on a Low Carb Lifestyle plan, let's discuss the good and bad fats. Many of the good fats that we will talk about and use in our recipes come in the form of butter, olive oil, coconut oil, peanut oil, lard, and as a byproduct of cream cheese, eggs, heavy cream, and animal fat. You will want to and need to avoid other fats that contain Transfats. Most of these transfats are found in such items as margarine, some vegetable shorting and oils. Later in this book we will talk about food labels and their importance. For now, when checking for transfats on products from the super markets shelves always check the ingredients for *partially hydrogenated.* Avoid the product, if you see this.

My two favorite cooking fats are clarified butter, which we will explain later in this book and good quality olive oil. An example of a good quality olive oil will be one that is labeled extra virgin. Extra virgin olive oil is known as the first extraction or cold extracted olive oil. These particular grades are preferred as they have no added chemicals and the first extraction, perseveres the fullest amount of vitamins and flavor. Often the extra virgin olive oils will add to the flavor of many of the dishes. In some cases you will find that I will suggest using a lesser grade of olive oil often combined with butter, for use in sautéing and high heat applications. When we want to experience or add the exceptional flavors from the extra virgin olive oil I will insist or specify in the recipe or directions that *"extra virgin olive oil"*, be used.

The following charts are of the oils and their uses that I may reference throughout this book.

OILS FOR SALAD

    Walnut oil
    Sesame Seed oil
    Peanut Oil

Olive Oil
Avocado Oil
Hazel Nut Oil
Almond Oil
Vegetable Oil (those not *partially hydrogenated)*

FATS FOR BAKING AND SAUTÉING

Butter
Clarified Butter (Ghee)
Coconut Oil
Olive Oil
Peanut Oil
Vegetable Oil (those not *partially hydrogenated)*
Lard

LOW CARB ON THE GO

Many busy individuals constantly struggle with upholding their Low Carb intake during their day. One thing I tell people is prepare as much of your own foods and snacks as possible. Here are but a few ideas that should help you through this if you are able to *"brown bag it"*. Egg salads, Chicken salad, Tuna salad, Shrimp salad, Turkey salad and Ham salad are but just a few of the homemade *"bound"* salads. You will find these recipes and suggestions later in the book. Also for the *"brown baggers"* consider a miniature deli tray of roast beef and cheese roll-ups, turkey and cheese roll-ups or ham and cheese roll-ups with olives a pickle spear and a cold drink and you will have a wonderfully satisfying lunch. Later in the book we will go into greater detail on the variations of these roll-ups. But now you say *"I don't have time for that, I always eat on the run"*. This I can always understand. For those of you that fall into that category here are my tips.

Don't let hectic days and travel sabotage your Low Carb Lifestyle. Here's how to navigate the high carb-laden landscape.

I know all too well that travel can make it harder to stay with the program. Suddenly, you're without your familiar routines and resources. Not only are you confronted with temptations you would never let into your house, you're exposed to them precisely when you're most vulnerable. If such reasons weren't risky enough, traveling in-and-of itself-can bring on stress, which in turn causes cravings for unhealthy foods.

So, what do you do? To succeed with the Low Carb Lifestyle, you must make a lifestyle change. That means dealing with every new circumstance in a way that is compatible with your commitment to new eating habits. When it comes to travel, the key to staying on track is a combination of mental and physical preparation. The following tips should help ensure that you don't leave your progress behind when you take your show on the road.

Think about your commitment. Don't use your trip as an excuse to go back to the old ways that caused the weight gain. Remember, if you continuously take detours from your planned route, you'll never reach your destination.

Take it with you. Pack some controlled-carb snack foods like ready to eat portions of cheese in plastic wrap. If you're traveling by car, pack a cooler with cold cuts and cheese or salad. Eat first. Start out on the right foot by eating a well-planned, satisfying meal before you leave.
Snack on nuts and seeds, which are high in protein and fat. You'll feel more satisfied and in control of your appetite after eating a handful.
No skipping allowed. Don't do it. Omitting a meal could make you ravenous, out of control and more likely to grab anything edible.
Drink up. Consume lots of water, which will help you feel satisfyingly full. But stay away from caffeine and diet sodas. These increase carbohydrate cravings.
Speed counts. If you do slip off for a day or more, get back on **AS SOON AS POSSIBLE**. The longer you're derailed, the harder it may be to get back on track.
Be ready to compromise without quitting. If you find all your food choices are poor, adhere to your Low Carb plan as closely as you can. For example, eat more salad and other vegetables. That doesn't mean

that you might as well eat bread and pasta. It's better to deviate a little than to toss the whole program out the window.

Finally, remember whose boss. You are in control of what goes in your mouth always, even when you're not in your own home. When dining out, ask how things are prepared and give instructions. After all, you're paying for it. Even in a fast-food restaurant, you're entitled to have it your way. Why should some stranger decide the success of your program, or your health?

Make Fast Food Friendly

Sandwich Shops: Chicken or tuna salad made with mayonnaise is a good choice. Just be sure to pick out any carrots. In sub shops, ask for the turkey, roast beef, cheese and sausage, but try to steer clear of salami, bologna and other meat products preserved with nitrates. Ask for your selection on a plate instead of on a roll.

Burger Chains: Sandwiches are usually a good bet. Just ignore the bun. Mayo and mustard are permissible but avoid the use of ketchup, which often contains a lot of sugar. Watch out too for special sauces, as they also often have sugar in them. Tomato slices and lettuce are fine. Steer clear of anything advertised as low-fat, an expression that often translates to high carb.

Fried Chicken Places: Avoid anything barbecued or breaded. Barbecue sauce is typically full of sugar and even if you remove the skin, the sugar has most likely leached into the meat. Dry-rubbed meats are fine, as are roasted chicken and allowed side dishes such as salad. If there's a grilled chicken filet sandwich available, grab it. Discard the bun, and you've got a good selection. Or scrape the breading off a fried chicken breast and include a salad for a complete lunch.

Salad Bars: Here you'll find the choices you need for a nutritious meal. Use olive oil and regular red or white wine vinegar instead of a prepared dressing. Commercial dressings and balsamic vinegars often contain sugar.

O k, so what did we just learn from all this? For many my hopes are a way to get through the day and for everyone to realize that *"this is not tough"*. **Just use common sense.**

T he real truth, the real strength behind all of what we've talked about and behind all of what I will share with you, is that first quote I introduced you to at the beginning *"nothing tastes as good as thin feels"*. I want each of you that read this book to implant that statement into your head. Now every time you look at a doughnut a bowl of pasta or any other non-allowed food, imagine that quote and get yourself to the point that just the mere thought of eating those foods troubles you with self-consumed guilt. Once you get to this point following the Low Carb Lifestyle becomes more common, more acceptable, and sensible with each passing day.

N obody but the late Dr. Atkins himself could possibly share more success stories and testimonials. However I assure you that of those that I supervised, inspired, and supported throughout the change from, high carb to a Low Carb Lifestyle, have come to live by that quote. And, I have seen those committed to themselves and their families lose thousands of pounds of unwanted fat.

LOW CARB TASTE GREAT

Let's remember that most of those Low Carb classical dishes we will explore will be the most satisfying dishes you may ever have. Why? Well let's look at some of the facts. After the first phase of the induction to Low Carb, most if not all of your cravings for high carb and sugar rich food will decrease or even disappear. Second, for most of you, any hunger attacks or *"hunger pains"* will also subside. So once these feelings and emotions subside, the days ahead will be filled with rich, robust and flavorful dishes. So now here is the beauty of this whole lifestyle of eating. The foods that you now will be eating will be higher in calories, for the most part, thus satisfying your caloric needs.

Second, eating fresh flavorful and rich meals also satisfies hunger much easier and for a longer period of time. Therefore I always insist that every effort be given to using only the finest ingredients available.

Think about something. How do you suppose it is that in most French Restaurants they can get by with the serving sizes you see? The answer is this, the food is rich in flavor and higher in calories from protein and fat. Therefore, your body is satisfied with the serving supplied. This will hold true with the meals we will learn here. Even those wonderful home style dishes we grew up with and adore, we will redo those here and be able to enjoy many of those same dishes.

I am told that one of the most challenging aspects of the culinary restrictions of this lifestyle is the change from all those high carb dishes most of us grew up with. Well truth be told, some of those will forever be banned from our lives on a daily basis until, as mentioned before, science and industry get on board the Low Carb train.

And you can trust in this, where there is demand and profits, industry will accommodate. That's the American way. Let's look at some of those Low Carb products now.

Nature's Own Reduced Carb Bread®. I have now found this in the 3 major supermarkets locally.

Steels Sugar free Fruit Pie Fillings®. I truly enjoy the new Steels Sugar free Fruit Pie Fillings. These make toppings for our Low Carb Cheesecake and other Low Carb treats. They're Splenda® sweetened, and come in four varieties: Apple, Peach, Cherry, and Blueberry.

LeCarb Frozen Dessert®. They're convenient little one-pint containers sugar free ice-creams that are sweetened with Splenda® and use glycerin to stay scoopable and of proper consistency. A regular serving is 1/2 cup and it comes in at 6 total carbs, with 3 of them being from glycerin, so if glycerin causes no reaction in you, count 3 carbs.

Mr. Freeze Freezer Pops®. Are Splenda® sweetened and come in about 1 carb per freezer pop. They come in boxes of 99 freezer pops, Blue Raspberry, Cherry, Lemon, and Grape. I have found these in several discount stores and wholesale/warehouse clubs, so look for them.

ThickenThin®. Non Starch Thickener, This is a pantry must. There are several trade names for this product such as, Thicken Up, Ready

Thick. You may have to mail order this item, as it is not as common on the supermarket shelves just yet.

Splenda®, of course is by far the closes to sugar on the market that is sugar free. This is but one of the products that will revolutionize the industry thinking about Low Carb.

Mt Olive®. New line of no sugar added pickles.

Pasta Although there are many alleged Low Carb pastas all over the net, this is the closes to the real thing. If you must have a replica Low Carb, this is the choice.
Darielle® http://web.inetba.com/jambsupplyinc/dariellepasta.htm

These Low Carb Tortillas are in a word, wonderful. I make use of these for many occasions.
Low Carb Tortillas® http://www.latortillafactory.com/index.htm

Every day now it seems a new product is offered in Low Carb, some are without question, very near to the "*real*" high carb original. However some, while they are a valiant effort, they are just not there yet. Mind you, as we have different pallets and likes and dislikes, many of the Low Carb commercially prepared products may well fit into your lifestyle. For my money and my particular likes, I have found the better quality products are being offered by the more well-known manufactures. Even still it is my choice to not tease myself with a "*near likeness*" of the real thing.

The few items listed above are but a small sampling of the Low Carb products now available. Some of which are in the recipes I have in this book, and will be mentioned throughout. This in no way should be considered a favored endorsement as should my exclusion of any product, not indicate my personal dislike of any product.

GETTING STARTED-MAKING THE CHANGE

By now I would trust most everyone reading this book has already either heard of or researched the many great benefits of the Low Carb Lifestyle. That being the case, I cannot and will not try to explain the scientific and medical dos and don'ts. Nor will I go into the hows and why this lifestyle works as well as it does. I will say from personal experience that it has changed my life and the lives of hundreds of people I have personally met since 1996. I will defer this to the Atkins center, as well as strongly recommend reading the late Dr. Atkins books in print on the subject. What I will do for you is install a mind-set and the confidence to make this a success. So here is my guide to getting started.

First and foremost, I will share with you the first thing I suggested to the staff at the Atkins center when I began working with them. "Hey don't you know diet is a four-letter word". We know from experience that diets never last a lifetime, and often are doomed from the beginning. For this to be a lifetime success we have to stop the diet thinking, using the word and address this as it is, a lifestyle. Just hearing the word diet is the first stage of anxiety. The second is trying to make sense of what most diets are expecting us to do, count measure and restrict every single morsel that passes our lips.

And the third strike is the failure to make enough noticeable changes to make the effort have any meaning. Let's face it, after several weeks of tedious counting calories, measuring, scooping and weighing, not to mention eating often tasteless "*Low Fat*" substitutes, little if any weight is lost. And worse yet, those jeans are still just as tight. We know changes in and of its self are tough, but with results starring us daily in the mirror, our jeans loosening up and eating rich full flavor foods, the change is much more tolerable. Until it, as I trust, will become your "*Lifestyle*". Now I already know what you're going to say, "*But we still have to count even on a Low Carb Lifestyle plan*". Well that's true to some extent, but in fact and in short time, you will see for yourself, your not counting, you're omitting unhealthy high carb food items. In fact, once you start thinking outside the box so-to-speak, you won't be counting at all. What you will be doing will become second nature to you, and in a short time you won't even have to give it a thought. You will be reprogrammed to eat, cook and order your food in a healthy Low Carb fashion day in day out.

So what can we conclude from all of this? Well like myself, I hope you can and do decide to make the change. Although it is not always easy, when we develop the proper mind-set and are given the moral support the resistance is reduced. Now throw in some "*I can't stand buying larger clothes every six months to a year*" (disgust), add to that a rich rewarding cuisine that corrects this, and you have one of the major keys to success. So now that that's all said, let us preview a few of the basics to getting started on a lifetime of change, a lifetime of success and looking and feeling better. The following tips are far from the whole picture of decadent cuisine and cooking. However, as we look at the many recipes I will explain how to achieve a balance between flavor, presentation and quality. So here are the beginning steps to a Low Carb cuisine.

LOW CARB COOKING TIPS

A lthough much contained on these pages may seem to be only common sense, I simply wish to reinforce these *"common sense"* items as well as share some new and fresh ideas with you that will make cooking the Low Carb Lifestyle as common as the every day cooking many of you have become used to.

1. Read and understand all packaged food labels. (we will discuss this much more)

2. Stock your pantry and refrigerator with plenty of Low Carb foods. (Clean out the bad foods.)

3. For breading a fried food make your own breading mixture from groundnuts and seasoning to taste.

4. Always use the freshest products available, there is no substitute for quality and flavor. A flavorful dish will satisfy your hunger and stop the want for snacks.

5. I like to teach students and professionals to *"build flavor"* as you go. By this always season and use fresh herbs and other Low Carb additions to your food items to again improve flavors. This is not a bland tasteless way to eat. Another example of adding flavor is

15

to use stocks in place of water wherever possible. Water is tasteless, whereas stocks add flavor.

6. **Reductions are your friend**. Always reduce stocks to improve flavor. Reduction is also the best choice for many soups and sauces to achieve a desired consistency in place of starch thickeners.

7. **Learn practice and perfect**: Learn to think Low Carb, practice cooking Low Carb and perfect your cooking skills. Many classical recipes that are some of the most flavorful and luxurious are naturally low in carbs. With a little practice you will learn to perfect these. A few examples are fresh mayonnaise from which you can make your own blue cheese dressing and Hollandaise Sauce from which you can make an endless array of great sauces. Let's not forget ice-cream. Think about it. Cream, eggs and sugar substitute (Splenda®) and a little flavoring agent and you have Low Carb ice-cream. Be creative. Once you set in place *"Low Carb"* thinking you will develop a flair for new food items to replace the common convenient junk food craving.

8. **Create**. Learn to create and pair food items so your meals don't have that *"I'm missing something"* look or taste to them. Blend different colors or textures on your plate. Arrange the foods to look nice, build height and above all keep variety in mind. Remember an Omelet isn't just for breakfast.

9. **Learn** to use purees of vegetables to create sauces, soups and thickeners. Pureed vegetables also make a great replacement for the traditional mashed potatoes. I often puree cauliflower add a little sour cream and butter with some horseradish. And guess what even my family thinks it is? Yes, Horseradish smashers!

10. **Experiment.** I have stumbled on some wonderful ways to replace many considered *"lost"* food items by saying *"what if"*. Here is an example. Would you believe you could make a California Roll

Low Carb? Guess what, you can, (and I do). So believe in yourself and get cooking…

11. **Be prepared.** One of the greatest excuses for failure in cooking is not being prepared. In a professional kitchen we refer to being prepared as having the mise en place in order. Defined, this means, to having all the ingredients necessary for a dish prepared and ready to combine up to the point of cooking. This is so important, especially in a home environment. It reduces tension and stress and reduces time as well. Again a successful action on our part ensures we will be more likely to continue our plan. So what does this means to you? First make certain you have all the needed ingredients, large and small. Have a well stocked pantry with seasonings, and condiments. Portion, cut, slice and or shape the food ahead of time. Have your cookware, bowls, cutting board and utensils nearby and ready to use. Clean as you go. Have clean towels, paper towels and rags nearby. Stay organized; don't let the scraps and product packaging pile up. Wash your utensils as you go. Keep your work area clean. And foremost be aware of any sanitation issues such as cross contamination. Work clean and work safe in your kitchen to avoid injuries and potential illness from improper food handling.

This may be the toughest of all tips for those of you with hectic lifestyles. Don't eat late at night. Try to allow at least 3, but preferable 4, hours before bedtime.

SHOPPING FOR LOW CARB

Reading Packaged Foods
NUTRITION LABELS

With today's busy schedules many people find it hard to prepare healthy meals. Fast-food restaurants are notorious for the high-fat, high-calorie, high-carbohydrate meals they offer.
Many people say they don't "*plan*" menus – at least they don't write them down in advance. But everyone plans, if only for how to stock the refrigerator or freezer.

"*P lanning menus*," means thinking about what foods to eat together for a meal, a day, or a week. Food choices are influenced by habit, by the occasion, by time and "*food available*" and by what you feel like eating, as well as by your concern for nutrition.

When shopping in accordance with your Low Carb Lifestyle, understanding the ratio of Carbohydrates-to-serving is essential in keeping your daily Carbohydrate intake low.

One important thing to know when selecting prepared food choices is how to read labels. That jargon on the label can be mysterious but it's important to learn what these terms mean in order to choose Low Carb foods. Here are those terms and their meanings:

Calorie Free – Fewer than 5 calories per serving.

Fat-Free – Less than 0.5g fat per serving.

Low Fat – 3 g (or less) of fat per serving.

Cholesterol Free – Less than 2 mg of cholesterol & 2 g (or less) of saturated fat per serving.

Low Cholesterol – 20 mg (or less) of cholesterol & 2 g (or less) of saturated fat per serving.

Very Low Sodium – 35 mg (or less) of sodium per serving.

Low Sodium – 140 mg (or less) per serving.

Sugar Free – Less than 0.5g of sugar per serving.

Low Carb – Less then 1.0g per serving.

No Carbohydrate – Less than 0.5g per serving. (Trace)

Serving Size: Serving size is set by the USDA and FDA. It is given in grams and household measures.

Calories & Calories from Fat: As well as total calories per serving, the label also lists how many of the calories come from fat.

Amount per Serving: Amount of a nutrient in one serving in grams or milligrams.

All packaged foods are required to carry a label with nutritional information for the consumer. The following are explanations of the items listed on these labels:

Side note: I have found when dedicating your lifestyle, to following a weight managing balance of Carbohydrates (as defined by Dr. Atkins) it is best to stock only *"Safe"* foods. By having the pantry and refrigerator stocked with recommended Low Carbs, what may appear as a challenge to eat only these foods is much easier to manage. The *"it was there"* thinking of food consumption is much less likely to have its way with you.

Now let's look at an example of one of these labels.

Nutrition Facts

Serving Size 4 cookies (31g)
Servings Per Container about 9

Amount Per Serving

Calories 160 | Calories from Fat 80

% Daily Value*

Total Fat 9g	13%
Saturated Fat 6g	28%
Cholesterol 0mg	0%
Sodium 140mg	6%
Total Carbohydrate 20g	7%
Dietary Fiber 1g	5%
Sugars 11g	
Protein 1g	

Vitamin A 0% • Vitamin C 0%

Calcium 0% • Iron 2%

* Percent Daily Values are based on a 2,000 calorie diet. Your daily values may be higher or lower depending on your calorie needs:

	Calories:	2,000	2,500
Total Fat	Less than	65g	80g
Sat Fat	Less than	20g	25g
Cholesterol	Less than	300mg	300mg
Sodium	Less than	2,400mg	2,400mg
Total Carbohydrate		300g	375g
Dietary Fiber		25g	30g

Calories per gram:
Fat 9 • Carbohydrate 4 • Protein 4

INGREDIENTS: ENRICHED FLOUR (WHEAT FLOUR, NIACIN, REDUCED IRON, THIAMINE MONONITRATE, RIBOFLAVIN), SUGAR, VEGETABLE SHORTENING (CONTAINS ONE OR MORE OF THE FOLLOWING PARTIALLY HYDROGENATED OILS: PALM KERNEL, SOYBEAN, COTTONSEED, COCOA (PROCESSED WITH ALKALI), CARAMEL COLOR, LEAVENING (SODIUM BICARBONATE, MONOCALCIUM PHOSPHATE, AMMONIUM BICARBONATE), HIGH FRUCTOSE CORN SYRUP, SALT, WHEY, SOY LECITHIN (EMULSIFIER), PEPPERMINT OIL, NATURAL AND ARTIFICIAL FLAVOR

Now using this label as an example what we first have to recognize is that this is obviously not a Low Carb food item. But more importantly what we have to consider is the serving size. Let's assume for a moment that you were considering the Carb value of this item in relationship to your serving. Notice in this case, the serving size is but Four (4) cookies, or 4 each. Ok we know we can't eat these items, in fact even if you subtract the one 1 gram of fiber included in the total carb count, you are still left with an alarmingly high 19 grams of Carbs for only 4 single cookies. Why is this important to us? One major common mistake I see all too often when helping individuals on a Low Carb Lifestyle is, understanding the relationship of portion size to Carb content. Notice after the actual Carb gram amount you will see 7%. This number can be misleading for, if you also notice, these allowed values are based on the FDA's 2000 calorie diet, which suggest 300 grams of Carbs, per day. This is dreadful! I don't consume 300 grams of Carbs in a week and neither will anyone following the Low Carb Lifestyle. Now here is the one obstacle with prepackaged foods. Many contain additives and usually some form of either sugar or various starches as a preservative or flavor enhancer (or worse yet to simply make the item look better during the canning or packaging process). Now, mind you, this does not mean that all canned or packaged items cannot be a part of the Low Carb Lifestyle but you must pay close attention to these labels.

Why am I making this point so strongly? Here is the bottom line. In many and most cases that serving size suggested on the label is smaller than what most people would consider by their standards. Second, and here is a real sore spot with me, many of the packaged Low Carb products and recipes in print and on the net in reality are simply a version of that re-created wheel I was talking about before. Yes these recipes and products often have a reduced Carb count. But if you look at the serving size in many cases, not all mind you, these are simply a smaller portion and therefore have a smaller Carb Count.

I'll share with you a prime example. A few years ago, here in the South Florida area, there was a local baker promoting he had created a *"true"* Low Carb fresh sliced sandwich style loaf of bread. Imagine my curiosity after seeing this advertisement. I found a local outlet for this bread and went to buy a loaf. Now here is what I found. First looking at his nutrition and ingredients label, the first thing I noticed was that this bread contained very near the same ingredients as in the typical commercial store-bought white bread. Oh sure he substituted a few percentages of product here and there with soy flour and a *"sugar substitute"*. But here is the real illusion. A typical slice of commercially produced sandwich style white bread indicates a single serving 1 slice as having after fiber subtraction a net 11 grams of Carbs. Also the typical slice being a serving size of roughly .9 ounces or just a pinch under 1 ounce in weight. The typical size of a slice of bread is roughly 4"x 41/2" and typically ¾" thick. Ok so why am I going into such boring detail about a single slice of bread? Well now watch. This Low Carb bread was less than half an ounce in weight and measured 3 1/2"x 3 1/2" and was just less than 3/8" in thickness; yes you could read a newspaper through it. Conclusion? Simple, this bread was no more Low Carb than a typical slice of *"Wonder Bread"* The only difference was that this baker had produced a loaf of miniature bread that cost nearly twice the price. Oh and it did not taste good at all.

So why would one tease themselves with this deceptive bread? It would make just as much sense to go to a local bakery, buy a typical loaf of pan white bread unsliced. Then take this loaf home and with my bread knife simply slice this bread paper-thin. Gee Low Carb. No, not really. Just a Low Carb serving. Do you see my point? This is a practice used commonly in both regular packaged food items and especially in the Low Carb product lines. Now is that sensible? So to go back a little, as I was pointing out before, until we have true Low Carb replacement products we either do without, or tease ourselves. In this case, having bought the real bread and sliced it to half its normal serving size I would have had half the Carbs, and all the taste.

So now that is the reason we will be describing true whole food in this book. There are plenty of readily available items to prepare wonder flavorful food items and menus. Now let's look at some tips for the types of products we will seek out.

I will say that it is always my preference and choice to use fresh products, be it, Produce, Meat, Fish and Chicken, etc. However there are times when for many reasons fresh either is not available or even less practical. When this is the case, I recommend products known as IQF, or individually quick-frozen. These products, when used according to directions, will serve nearly identical as fresh in most recipes. Often it is just not practical to buy fresh. A few good examples of this would be IQF Chicken Wings, IQF Fish Fillets, and IQF Shrimp. As for produce you can often find IQF Broccoli, IQF whole and cut Green Beans and IQF Cauliflower. Now I mention these items simply because in many cases, especially with seafood, these items are less in price than fresh and in many recipes these IQF products are perfectly suitable. Often we also see these IQF items packaged and sold in sizes that make them a great value. They also store well until needed. Finally you can use what numbers you need since these are frozen individually and return the rest back to the freezer for later use. Now let's take some time to review how to recognize quality in the products that we will commonly be using in many of the dishes in this book. Use the following guidelines when shopping for these products. I want to once again emphasis the importance of good quality products. There is no substitute for quality.

QUALITY GUIDELINES

BEEF

When shopping for beef or veal in most retail supermarkets you will typically see one or two grades of beef. These are established by the USDA and they indicate the amount of marbling or fat in the meat. The three most common grades are Prime, Choice and Select. Prime being the most marbled, resulting in a more flavorful and tender cut of beef. Typically this grade is seldom seen in most retail supermarkets. As the cost is notably higher as well as much of this grade of beef goes to processors supplying those Prime Steak Houses, Country Clubs and the high-end beef business. This is not to say your local market doesn't carry Prime, and if the price is right buy it.

Choice beef is by far the most commonly sold beef in the retail market. When buying choice beef always look for a nice marbling throughout the beef. We now see more Blank Angus Choice Beef, and if your market carries this line and the cost is not considerably higher, I will recommend buying Black Angus Beef. However, the better cuts of choice will and do cook and taste just fine. Select Beef is the least marbled of the three grades, meaning less fat, flavor and often a tougher cut of beef. Typically these cuts are also less moist. Nowadays more of the portion cut beef selections are vacuum-packaged. I always prefer to buy products packaged in this fashion if it's an item I am not going to use within two days. The advantage is that because of the lack of oxygen the product has a much longer shelf life and, in fact the beef tends to continue to tenderize as it sits.

While on the subject, I have a home vacuum packaging system. I bought this item for under $75.00. The great advantage to this is when those deals are out there; you can buy in volume take your product home and package it in sizes that serve your needs. The huge advantage is longer shelf life, and little or no chance of freezer burn. This works well even for fresh produce.

What to Look For;

Select beef with a bright cherry-red color, without any grayish or brown blotches. The exception is vacuum-packaged beef which, in the absence of oxygen, has a darker purplish-red color; when exposed to the air, it will turn to a bright red.

Look for beef that is firm to the touch, not soft.

Make sure the package is cold and has no holes or tears.

Choose packages without excessive liquid.

For highest quality, always check and buy beef before the sell-by date.

Retail Cuts of Beef

Butchering techniques and the names and shapes of cuts differ from area to area. However, one point of agreement is that the best (and most expensive) cuts come from the back half of the animal, especially from the fleshy hindquarters (the loin, sirloin and round).

Top-quality cuts respond best to cooking in dry heat, such as grilling, roasting and pan-frying:

Tenderloin. The most tender cut. The tenderloin, or fillet, is the strip of flesh inside the rib cage that runs parallel to the spine. The thinnest part of the tenderloin is used for filets mignons and the wide end can be used for châteaubriand. T-bone steaks are the end of the sirloin and a piece of the tenderloin.

Rump. Part of the round; rump roast and steaks with tough tendons that should be removed with a sharp knife. Steaks from this section are usually juicy and can be cooked with dry heat methods. Rump roasts are usually cooked using moist heat.

Rib. Consists of ribs 6 thru 12 and a portion of the backbone. Cuts include rib roast, blade, short ribs, rib-eye roast and rib-eye steaks.

Round (topside or silverside in Britain) meat cut from the hind leg; divided into top round, eye of round and bottom round; may be cut into steaks, but mostly used for boneless roasts. These cuts are usually tender and flavorful. Top round is lean and good for pot-roasting.

Flank. The area beneath the loin and behind the short plate. The meat has a coarse texture and plenty of fat; flavorful but tough. Flank steak is often used for London broil. Skirt steak also comes from this region.

Sirloin tip. Top sirloin (top rump or thick flank in Britain) boneless cut from the top round; makes excellent pot roast or can be cubed for stews.

Brisket. The animal's breast section between the foreshank and short plate; boneless, tough but flavorful.

Chuck (bladebone in Britain) the shoulder area including ribs 1 thru 5 and some of the backbone; juicy and flavorful. Chuck is used for cubed steak, chuck roast and ground beef.

Foreshank. The animal's foreleg; good for stews but needs long, slow cooking.

POULTRY

Poultry for our purpose here will include chicken, whole or cut, squab, duck, turkey, Cornish hens, rabbit and goose. Here are some great tips about poultry.

Buying poultry

You can buy poultry in any form you want. Chicken can be bought whole, cut into halves or quarters, boneless, sliced (breasts or thighs) or cubed. You can buy chicken from the butcher shop or from the supermarket. Whole or cut chicken bought from the butcher shop should be cleaned and all inner parts removed. You can also ask the poultryman to remove its bones, or cut it into any form you want. If you buy chicken from the supermarket, make sure there is no liquid at the bottom of the package plate. Also avoid packages that are torn, not well frozen, or have an off smell. Turkey, pigeons, and duck are usually sold whole. Rabbit is usually cut into pieces but if you need it for stuffing or roasting, have the poultryman leave it as a whole

Gregory Pryor C.E.C.

Storing poultry

You can keep poultry in the fridge (cooked or uncooked) for a maximum 2 days. Make sure it is well wrapped and closed tightly.

Washing and cleaning poultry

Whole chicken should be bought cleaned with all the inner parts removed. If there are any parts left, remove them. Soak for 10-15 minutes in cold water with salt and/or vinegar. Take some salt and rub chicken well both inside and outside with it using your hands. Rinse well under running water. Repeat until chicken is cleaned. If it still smells, rub the inside with a lemon half. With a sharp knife remove any excess fat or small bones that you will not use.

Rabbit and pigeon are washed in the same way. Whole turkey is washed in the same way, but make sure it is well cleaned when buying it. In a case of duck, rub it with more salt and make sure the skin is smooth and doesn't contain the roots of any feathers. Cut chicken: Wash well under running water. Don't wash chicken or soak it in hot water. This changes its color and makes the blood clot inside the meat.

Freezing and defrosting poultry

In case of whole poultry, rinse with water and remove any parts that you don't use. Leave to drain well in a colander. In other cases, don't wash. Put on foam plates covered with plastic wrap or in plastic bags. Remove excess air, close well and place in the freezer. Freeze up to 3-5 months. Cooked poultry can stay frozen up to 1-month.

To defrost, take it out of the freezer and leave it in the fridge overnight. Put it in a dish or another plastic bag to contain the liquid that it releases. You can also soak it, wrapped, in cold water. Don't run hot water over it or soak it in it. This changes its color and makes the blood clot inside the meat.

PORK

Buying fresh pork is not a difficult process, and you should feel comfortable when deciding about specific cuts. When buying pork, the key qualities to look for are: cuts with a small amount of fat on the outside, firm looking composition, and a pink to red color. Selecting pork with these qualities will assure you that your eating experience will be enjoyable. When buying pork, look for meat that's pale pink with a small amount of marbling and white (not yellow) fat. The darker pink the flesh, the older the animal.

Store fresh pork that will be used within 6 hours of purchase in the refrigerator in its store packaging. Otherwise, remove the packaging and loosely wrap with plastic wrap; store in the coldest part of the refrigerator for up to 2 days. Ground pork and pork sausage shouldn't be stored for more than 1 or 2 days.

Pork can be frozen for 3 to 6 months; larger cuts have longer storage capabilities than chops or ground meat.

Gregory Pryor C.E.C.

Retail Cuts of Pork

All cuts of pork can be satisfactorily roasted, as the pig does not develop much tough muscle or connective tissue. It is important to cook all cuts thoroughly.

Leg. Often boned and divided into the shank or leg end and the butt end or top leg (called fillet in Britain). Boned, rolled shank is easier to cook evenly; however, when cooking shank on the bone, you can protect the thinner bony section by wrapping it in aluminum foil halfway through the cooking process. Leave the meatier end exposed to full heat. Cook the butt end, boneless or not, as a roast. Or slice into ¼- to 1-inch thick cutlets and prepare as steak. The butt end can also be cut into cubes for kebabs.

Loin. The tender, delicate meat from this section is excellent boned, stuffed, rolled and roasted. The fleshy sirloin is usually cut into thick chops (called sirloin or butterfly chops), or thick sirloin cutlets. Rib or loin chops can be pan-fried, broiled or braised. Back ribs also come from this section (baby back ribs are simply from younger animals and are smaller). Country-style ribs are the thick, meaty ribs from the shoulder end of the loin.

Spareribs. From the lower section of the rib cage; usually sold in slabs and prepared by barbecuing. Very bony with little meat, so allow at least 1½ pounds per person.

Tenderloin. Usually sold vacuum-packed in plastic; lean and tender. Whole tenderloin can be roasted or grilled. Tenderloin has a delicate flavor.

Shoulder. Often called Boston butt; picnic ham, blade roasts and steaks come from this section. The rich meat can be roasted or ground for sausage. Steaks are good for barbecuing over charcoal.

Side. Also called the belly; this section provides bacon and other fatty meat that is usually cured.

PRODUCE

Select fresh produce with rich color that is firm to the touch to measure freshness and vitamin content. The richer the color the higher the nutrient content.

Beware of bruises, soft spots, cuts, wrinkles, discolored areas and surface breaks. These are signs that it has passed its peak of freshness. A smaller vegetable often indicates it has more flavor and a tender texture.

Asparagus should be firm and have straight stalks with closed tips.
Broccoli should have rich, green, firm buds that are packed closely together. Slender stalks mean tender florets.
Cabbage – Pick heads that feel heavy with tender leaves of rich color.
Cauliflower should be creamy white with bright green leaves. Pick heavy solid heads.
Celery should be crisp, firm and unblemished. Leaves should be fresh and green, not yellow and droopy.
Eggplant should have a deep purple smooth skin free of scars and cuts. It should be heavy and firm.
Green beans should be straight, long and snap when bent.
Lettuce – Pick heads that feel heavy with tender leaves of rich color.
Mushrooms should be firm and plump and have closed caps.

Gregory Pryor C.E.C.

Onions should be firm with short necks and have paper like outer skins.
Peppers should be firm, smooth and glossy.
Tomatoes should be free of cracks and bruises.

FRESH HERBS

Nothing excites me more than a nice variety of fresh herbs. These wonderful flavored herbs can add so many dimensions to many of the dishes we will prepare. With the fresh herbs we will make flavored butters and improve soups, stocks and sauces. We will create herb crust on roasted meats, make dry rubs and add color and presentation to our dishes. Here are a few tips for fresh herbs.

Basil Traditionally used on tomatoes, whether cooked or raw. In salads, basil's leaves and tender stems give a sweet and mildly pungent flavor to various other foods. It is especially fine on lamb chops, in cheese dishes, with peas and string beans.

Prep: Pull leaves from stems and wash well. Use whole or freshly chopped.

Garlic. Sections of bulb, whole, chopped or crushed. Strong, pungent, penetrating; to be used with discretion.

Parsley. The most popular herb. Several varieties. Fragrant and flavorful. Comes tightly curled or with pungent flat leaves (sometimes called Italian parsley). The main herb in bouquet garni and is fine for seasoning meat. Sprigs and leaves usually used fresh, but dried leaves are available. Aromatic; contains minerals and vitamin C.

Prep: Pull the leaves from the coarse stems and wash well. (Stems can be used too.)

Tip: Chop a whole bunch of parsley at one time, then freeze what you don't need right away. Or wrap in a white paper towel and a plastic bag. It will keep several days in the refrigerator.

Rosemary. Mostly a meat herb, rosemary is the leaf of an evergreen shrub and shaped like a curved pine needle. It has a sweet flavor and bitter taste fresh from the garden than when dried. It is excellent with lamb, fish and poultry.

Prep: Run fingers down stems against the growth to remove leaves. Chop spiny leaves.

Tarragon. Best known as a flavoring agent for Béarnaise Sauce and vinegar. Tarragon is good in seafood. Both the dried leaves and the flowering tops may be used for the faintly anise-like flavor.

Prep: Remove the long tender leaves off the stems before chopping.

Thyme. The finest herb for fish and shellfish soups, like clam chowder and oyster stew. Thyme may be sprinkled in the cooking water of a lobster or add to a poultry dressing. One of the most versatile culinary herbs. Thyme is aromatic and pungent, and goes well with tomatoes, fricassees and chipped beef.

Prep: Remove the tiny leaves from the woody stems before chopping. Easiest way is to run two fingers over the stems, top to bottom.
Now let's look at some suggestions for a well stocked pantry.

My pantry at home would by most people's thinking seem rather *"busy"* or perhaps to some overstocked. However I can say honestly nearly every item in my pantry is used regularly. So starting with the basics and moving along, in my pantry you will find these items. Salt, several types; Sea Salt, Course Kosher Salt, and of course the typical table salt. I also have the typical seasoned salt, of which I make huge use of for seasoning many dishes. Pepper, again many varieties, course ground black pepper, mixed ground pepper, several different peppercorn blends, dried pepper flakes, cayenne pepper, and of course fine ground black pepper. Also you will find many dried herbs, rosemary, thyme, tarragon, paprika, cumin, oregano, turmeric, saffron and any other dried herbs and seasoning that you individually enjoy. You will find also Splenda®. ThickenThin®, Chili Oil, Olive Oils, Peanut Oil, Lard, Various whole and sliced nuts and of course cornstarch and flour, although rarely used and in limited quantity when I do use these. Each of you should tailor your pantry to your own style of cooking and of course to the limits you may have in respect to size. Again your pantry will take on a look and stock of items as you become more accustomed to *"thinking outside the box"* in respect to your Low Carb Lifestyle. I simply enjoy having a well stocked pantry so when I decide to do a dish, say like a Southwestern spice rubbed rack of lamb, I have the ingredients to complete the dish with little or no special shopping time involved. Another key addition to your kitchen area is a quality set of *"Sharp"* knives. Do you know more people are harmed or injured using a dull knife than one of good sharp quality? Do you know why? When you use a dull ill fitting knife you will have a tendency to 1. Grip the knife in an unsafe manner and 2. Apply greater pressure when making cuts, often causing the item to move or the knife to slip under such added effort. Proper knife skills are essential to work safely and efficiently in the kitchen.

As well as a good set of knives, you will also need a good solid, heavy cutting board. I have no problem at all with the typical hard plastic type, as long as they are of good size and weight. A little tip when using these type cutting boards, especially on a home countertop or work surface. Place a wet kitchen towel or even a damp paper towel under the board to prevent it from sliding on the work surface and, again, prevent further injury. I like to have several of these around so I can use one for cutting raw items and another for cutting produce or other items. Produce should never come in contact with uncooked raw items such as meats, chicken, fish etc.

Gregory Pryor C.E.C.

A nother question, I am often asked is, "What small kitchen appliances should I have?" Wow, am I the wrong one to ask! For my thinking I love gadgets, so I say *"have them all"*. However, I know that is not practical and often not feasible for each of us. So my answer is this, the two most commonly used small kitchen appliances we will use are a good food processor and a stand type mixer or *"Kitchen Aide®"*. I use these two items more than any other small appliance you could find in our home. The processor is a valuable tool when we look at making for example, groundnuts or mixed dried herbs for spice rubs and seasonings. They're great for fine chopping vegetables or garlic using a pulsed action. Many of the salad dressings are a snap to prepare in the food processor. For example, Caesar, Green Goddess and Mayonnaise based dressings and spreads can be made in a snap. Flavored mayonnaise is one of my favorite additions to many dishes to add flavor and moisture. The Kitchen Aide is another nearly essential appliance in that with this we mix the batter things like cheesecake. We whip our eggs for custards and make whipped cream for desserts and with the food grinder attachment we can grind our own ham for ham salad. I now even grind my own no-sugar-added pickles to make various types of relishes and condiments. I feel like I could write a book solely on the kitchen and its components. But for sake of discussion, as we talk about a recipe or dish that I feel would benefit from the mention of a special appliance use or kitchen tool I will do so in the recipe or dish conversation. Now having said all this, LET'S START COOKING!

O k first in our line of Low Carb recipes I want to talk about appetizers. The following are some principles used when we consider appetizers. These guidelines will help you in understanding appetizers. Mind you, much of this content is not solely for the purpose of Low Carb items. However, as you will discover, much of the principle is the same. What we do is take these principles and apply our *"outside the box"* Low Carb Thinking to them to create a varied array of Low Carb appetizers. Please understand when I outline throughout this book any principles, I am doing so for general culinary procedures and guides. By doing so I hope that *"you"* will gain the knowledge and thinking to apply Low Carb techniques to all your cooking needs.

APPETIZERS

Hors d'oeuvre: is a French term whose translation is *"outside the work"* which means small tidbits served apart from the main meal. While the term appetizer and hors d'oeurve are often used interchangeably in this country, generally an appetizer is the first course of a multicourse meal while finger foods served at receptions and with cocktails are referred to as hors d'oeuvre. Traditionally, it was the service staff who prepared hors d'oeuvre while the kitchen staff prepared the meal.

Guidelines for preparing Hors d'oeurve:
They should be small, 1 to 2 bites.
They should be flavorful and well seasoned without being overpowering.
They should be visually attractive.
They should compliment the foods to follow without duplicating flavors.

CANAPÉS – are tiny open-faced sandwiches.
There are four components to a canapé:
The base
The spread

The topping or main item
The garnish

The Base:

The most common base is a thin slice of bread cut into an interesting shape. If the bread is soft, it is usually toasted. If it is a firmer variety such as pumpernickel, it is sometimes used untoasted.

The base must be strong enough to support the weight of the spread and topping without falling apart.

When selecting a base for a canapé it is important to consider the flavor of all the components and how they will interact with one another. Since bread is not always the best choice for us, consider this. Use cucumber sliced 1½ inch thick, scoop out a small section in the center and fill this with any number of fillings. Or consider halved Roma tomatoes, again filled with any number of fillings. Medium and large cherry tomatoes also make a wonderful canapé when hollowed out and filled.

The Spread:

The spread provides much of the canapé's flavor. Spreads may be used either as a substantial portion of the canapé or used sparingly as a means of gluing on the topping and garnish.

The most common spreads are flavored butters, cream cheese or a combination of the two.

Another especially good spread to use for a Low Carb version is flavored mayonnaise.

Guidelines for making spreads:

The texture should be smooth enough to produce an attractive design if piped.

The consistency should be firm enough to hold it's shape, yet soft enough to stick to the base and hold toppings an/or garnishes.

The spreads flavor should complement the topping and garnish but not be overpowering.

Canapés with bread bases tend to get soggy quickly from both the moisture in the bread as well as moisture from the refrigerator. Three ways to combat this are:
Using spreads made with butter.
Spreading the base with a thin layer of plain butter before piping on a spread.
Make as close to service as possible.

The Topping:

The topping or main item of a canapé is any food item or combination of items placed on top of the spread. It is the major part of a canapé, such as a slice of smoked salmon or a coronet of salami.
Items used for the topping should be of a consistent size and shape.

The Garnish

The garnish of a canapé adds eye appeal. It should enhance the canapé.
The varieties of garnishes used are limitless; however, the overall flavor and look of the canapé should be the deciding reason when selecting garnishes.

Butter Recipes: When making the following recipes, keep in mind the following points:
Use only high quality unsalted butter.
Before adding other ingredients, bring butter to room temperature.
All ingredients mixed with the butter should be pureed or as with herbs finely chopped to make a smooth product.
All the below recipes are made with 1 pound of butter.
After ingredients are added to the butter, the butter should be mixed until it is smooth.

Gregory Pryor C.E.C.

To 1# of Butter Add
Type
Anchovy   2 oz pureed anchovy fillets
Blue Cheese   4 oz pureed blue cheese
Chive   1 bunch chives, minced
Garlic   2 cloves pureed garlic
Horseradish   4 oz horseradish
Lemon   4 T lemon juice & 2 T zest
Lobster   12 oz pureed cooked lobster
Mint   6 tsp finely chopped mint
Onion   1 small Spanish onion, minced
Pimento   8 oz pureed pimentos
Shrimp   12 oz pureed cooked shrimp
Salmon   8 oz. pureed smoked or cooked salmon
Tuna   8 oz of pureed canned squeezed dry tuna

Once you have the butter will mixed, use either a large piece of parchment paper, waxed paper or plastic wrap, spread the butter on any one of these and roll into a log. Roll up tightly and twist the ends to make an even sized roll. Now you can store this butter either in the fridge or freezer to use as needed. Typically I have several various flavored or compound butters, as I use these nearly in every dish I prepare.

Flavored Mayonnaise
Here are some easy, flavorful spreads, all based on store-bought Mayonnaise.

Roasted Garlic Mayonnaise

Makes about 1 1/4 cups

For roasted garlic

1 whole garlic head

1 tablespoon olive oil

For mayonnaise

1 cup mayonnaise

Fresh lemon juice to taste

Salt and freshly ground black pepper

Roast garlic: Preheat oven to 350 degrees F. Place head of garlic on piece of foil, drizzle with 1 tablespoon olive oil, and tightly wrap. Bake until tender, about 45 minutes; cool slightly. Squeeze garlic from skin into bowl and mash lightly with fork.

Garlic mayonnaise: Add 1 cup mayonnaise, fresh lemon juice, and salt and pepper to roasted garlic pulp and stir to combine.

Basil Mayonnaise
Makes 1 1/4 cups

1 cup mayonnaise

1/2 cup loosely packed fresh basil leaves, rinsed and patted dry.

Salt and freshly ground black pepper to taste.

In blender or food processor, combine all ingredients and blend until smooth. Transfer to bowl for serving.

Mustard Chive Mayonnaise
Makes about 1 1/4 cups

The ideal spread for canapés of roast beef, baked ham, pastrami, or corned beef, paired with cheeses like Swiss or Provolone.

1 cup mayonnaise

2 tablespoons sour cream

Gregory Pryor C.E.C.

1 to 2 tablespoons Dijon mustard

2 tablespoons snipped fresh chives or scallion tops

Salt to taste

In bowl combine all ingredients.

Here are a few ideas for making canapés.

Using Natures Own Low Carb bread, cut rounds of the bread using a small one-inch pastry cutter. After cutting as many rounds from each slice as needed for the number of canapés you wish to prepare, toast these on a cookie sheet in a 350 degree oven. Turn to brown lightly each side and use the following as examples. By the way, you should get 4-5 rounds per slice, with a net carb of less than .5 gram per round. Now let's suppose we would like to make a simple roast beef and cheese canapé. Prepare the Mustard Chive Mayonnaise and set aside. Use the same pastry cutter as you did to cut the bread and cut the same number and size rounds of the roast beef and your favorite cheese, (in this case I would use cheddar). Lightly spread the flavored mayonnaise on each round of bread. If you want a taller and more substantial canapé simply continue to stack the roast beef and cheese one atop each other. Finally, I would garnish the top with a tiny snip of chive in a tiny drop of the mayonnaise to secure the garnish. Now using this principle you can change these or add a mix using Ham and Swiss, and a flavored horseradish mayonnaise. Have a few more thoughts and ideas? I hope so. Suppose you wanted a cream cheese and smoked salmon canapé. That's simple: Using the same bread rounds simply beat some room temperature cream cheese. Spread a light amount on the bread, then using any prepackaged sliced smoked salmon, gently roll each slice up and sit it on the spread. A great garnish would be a tiny drop of the spread and a caper or a piece of red onion on top. So, do you see where I am going with these ideas? You as well can create an endless array of canapés from the basics provided here. Also, later along in the book of recipes you will find many dips and *"bound salads"* (those made typically with mayonnaise) that can also make a topping for canapés.

Now let's look at some other types of appetizers. The more likely ones we would see and prepare for ourselves for use at home. For example, Bacon wrapped scallops, Chicken Satay with peanut sauce, Swedish meatballs, Chicken nuggets and who could overlook deviled eggs. The variety of deviled eggs should never allow you to grow tired of these wonderful appetizers. Just stop and consider for a minute all the varieties of the filling and garnish you can add to typical deviled eggs. Consider a little curry powder to the typical egg yolk and mayonnaise mixture. Or try adding a little pickle relish, made from the new Mt. Olive® *"no sugar added"* pickles. You can feel free to add this with no worries of increasing the carb count. Garnish each with a caper, or a tiny slice of black olive. One of my favorite garnishes is to add a tiny dollop of fish eggs, or inexpensive caviar. Another favorite is Baked Brie with Toasted Almonds. This is a very easy and fast appetizer to prepare. Simply brush any size wheel of Brie with egg whites, scatter some sliced blanched almonds over-the-top and bake until the cheese just begins to run. Remove and let stand 10 minutes before serving. The ideas could be endless once you expand your Low Carb thinking.

Another of my favorite appetizers, and one that we can enjoy with almost no guilt or Carb concerns at all, are roll-up pinwheels. Let's talk about this a bit. These items are near and dear to the Low Carb Lifestyle. They can serve as a wonderfully easy lunch item replacement for the typical High Carb sandwich. These can be expanded to be used as a tray of appetizers served alongside deviled eggs, or even a tray of crudité and dip. Let's look at some examples from simple to elegant. A simple example, and one I use often for my lunch, simply uses any of the following meats: Sliced roast beef, turkey or ham. To each slice of any of these simply lay a piece of sliced cheese and roll them up. How much easier could this be? This also satisfies that need for a lunch time sandwich, especially when you add a pickle spear and a serving of cottage cheese. It is a complete lunch. And the great part is, you can have as many of these at you like, because they are almost carb free. Now let's look at another example that makes a wonderful platter item. What I do is this; I buy for example one pound each roast beef, turkey breast and ham. I then buy a quarter pound of 2 or 3 different sliced cheeses from the deli. For example, a sharp cheddar, an aged Swiss and one of my favorites, hot pepper cheese. Now to assemble these for appetizer use, follow these suggestions and feel free to adapt to your own preferences.

First, before we go into the details of this appetizer, picture in your mind the typical High Carb wrap, or sandwich roll often made with flat bread. Now that we can picture this in our mind, let's create our healthy Low Carb version. Now, here is how we do this. For each roll take a slice of each deli meat item. Now working either on a clean work surface or a large cutting board, lay each piece side by side with each slightly overlapping the other. Once you have this stage completed, spread a thin layer of either mayonnaise, mustard or any of the flavored mayonnaise mixtures offered in this book, (or make one that is to your preference). Add the cheese of your choice. Now we can continue to build our roll. Next lay some lettuce over the spread, such as Bibb lettuce, butter lettuce or leaf. Be certain to choose a lettuce that is thin leafed and pliable. Even the larger outer leaves of iceberg will work for this product. If you like, at this point you can continue with other condiments such as pickle chips or thin sliced spears, tomato slices, chopped black olives or any other Low Carb item that you would like. Now repeat the meat cover only in reverse order of the items to create a contrast. Lightly season this with salt and pepper. Then in a jelly roll fashion roll this up firmly, taking care not to tear the meat yet tight enough to stay together. Once you have the roll complete and laying before you in a long even cylinder, cut each roll into 1½ inch thick slices on a bias. Continue the preparation for as many of these roll up pinwheels that you may need to create your deli roll up platter. Imagine how nice and complete your appetizer table will look with a platter of crudité and dip, deviled eggs with various garnishes and these attractive and flavorful pinwheels.

The following recipes should provide you with a variety of ideas to further you're thinking about the Low Carb possibilities.

Appetizers

Bacon-Wrapped Scallops
Servings: 24

24 sea scallops, about 2 pounds
12 slices bacon
Seasoned salt and pepper

Cook bacon gently until partially cooked but not crisp and still flexible. Rinse scallops with running cold water, pat dry with paper towels. Cut each bacon slice crosswise in half; wrap each half around a scallop, securing with a toothpick. Sprinkle scallops lightly with salt and pepper. Preheat broiler. Place scallops on rack in broiling pan.
Broil 4 to 5 inches from heat for 8 to 10 minutes, or until scallops turn opaque throughout, using tongs to turn scallops often so bacon will brown evenly on all sides.

Nutrition per Serving
Carbs: 1 g Fiber: 0 g **Net Carbs: 1 g** Protein: 2 g Fat: 12.5 g Calories: 9

Gregory Pryor C.E.C.

Appetizers

Chicken Nuggets

Servings: 20

3 tablespoons ThickenThin®
1 teaspoon salt
1/2 teaspoon Splenda®
2 tablespoons dry sherry
2 egg whites
1 whole chicken breast, cut into 1-inch pieces
3/4 cup hazelnuts, dry-roasted, finely chopped or Macadamia nuts
Oil for frying

MUSTARD SAUCE
1/4 cup mayonnaise
1 tablespoon dry mustard
1/4 teaspoon Splenda®

Combine ThickenThin®, salt and Splenda®. Stir in sherry. Beat egg whites until foamy. Stir in ThickenThin® mixture. Dip chicken in mixture and roll in nuts, pressing nuts into chicken. Place on rack to dry. Fry in hot oil until done. Drain and serve with a mustard sauce, if desired.
For Mustard Sauce: Blend all ingredients together and serve.

Nutrition per Serving
Carbs: 1 g Fiber: 0 g **Net Carbs: 1 g** Protein: 7 g Fat: 12.5 g Calories: 88

Appetizers

Cheese and Sausage Nuggets

Servings: 36

Almond meal is prepared by pulsing blanched sliced Almonds in a food processor till very fine, almost like flour.

8 eggs
1/2 cup almond meal
1 teaspoon baking powder
3/4 teaspoon salt
3 cups Mozzarella cheese
1 1/2 cups cottage cheese
3/4 pound spicy pork sausage, cooked and crumbled

In large bowl, beat eggs, add almond meal, baking powder and salt. Blend thoroughly. Fold in remaining ingredients. Turn into a greased 9 × 9 × 2-inch baking dish. Bake in a 350ºF oven for 40 minutes. Remove from oven; let stand 10 minutes. Cut into small squares; serve warm or at room temperature.

Nutrition per Serving
Carbs: 1 g Fiber: 0 g **Net Carbs: 1 g** Protein: 2 g Fat: 12.5 g Calories: 100

Appetizers

Firehouse Red Stuffed Mushrooms
Servings: 16

For this recipe raw clean white mushrooms are fine, however by slightly cooking the mushrooms, we improve the flavor.
To prepared cooked mushrooms, carefully remove the stems; wipe each mushroom with a damp paper towel.
Take a sharp paring knife and take a small slice off each cap to create a flat base so the mushroom to sit flat. After all mushrooms are cleaned and cut, season each with salt and pepper then sit each cavity side down on a baking screen placed over a cookie sheet. Place in a 350 degree oven and cook till mushrooms give off their liquid and turn slightly brown, but not wilted. About 10-15 minutes. Remove, cool and continue to filling each.
Let cool in refrigerator 1-hour before service.

1 8-ounce package cream cheese, softened
1/4 cup Roasted Red Pepper, patted dry
2 tablespoons grated Parmesan cheese
1 teaspoon minced garlic
1 Pinch ground red pepper
1 pound medium-size fresh white mushrooms

Remove stems from mushrooms; reserve caps; save stems for mushroom soup or other use.
See tips above how to prepare mushrooms for stuffing.
In a bowl of a food processor with a metal blade, place cream cheese, roasted red peppers, Parmesan cheese, garlic and ground red pepper. Process until smooth, about 1-minute.
In a pastry bag fitted with a large star tip, place cream cheese mixture. Pipe into mushroom caps; garnish with toasted pine nuts, sliced green olives and parsley leaves, if desired.

Nutrition per Serving
Carbs: 2 g Fiber: 1 g **Net Carbs: 1 g** Protein: 2 g Fat: 5 g Calories: 60

Appetizers

Cheese Topped Mushrooms
Servings: 24

To prepare mushrooms, carefully remove the stems; wipe each mushroom with a damp paper towel. Take a sharp paring knife and take small slice off each cap to create a flat base for the mushroom to sit flat.

1 pound bulk pork sausage
1 pound fresh mushrooms, about 24 each (medium to large mushroom work best)
1 clove garlic, finely minced
2 tablespoons chopped parsley
1 1/2 cups shredded Cheddar cheese (6 ounces)
Chopped pimiento (optional)
Fresh snipped parsley (optional)

Wipe mushrooms with a damp towel and pat dry; remove stems. Chop stems. Combine stems, sausage, garlic and chopped parsley in a medium skillet; cook until sausage is browned, stirring often. Drain pan drippings. Stir in cheese, mixing well.
Fill mushroom caps with sausage mixture. Place in a 13 × 9 × 2-inch baking dish. Bake at 350°F for 20 minutes.
Garnish with pimiento and snipped parsley, if desired.

Nutrition per Serving
Carbs: 1 g Fiber: 0 g **Net Carbs: 1 g** Protein: 1 g Fat: 1 g Calories: 5

Gregory Pryor C.E.C.

Appetizers

Crab-Stuffed Mushrooms
Servings: 24

Shrimp can be substituted for crab.

1 cup cooked flaked crab meat, canned and picked clean is fine.
8 ounces cream cheese, softened
1 teaspoon lemon juice
2 Dashes Worcestershire sauce
1/4 teaspoon basil
1/4 teaspoon garlic powder
2 green onions, minced
1/8 teaspoon lemon pepper
24 large mushrooms
1/2 cup Cheddar cheese, grated
2 tablespoons freshly grated Parmesan cheese

Wash mushrooms well, remove stems, and set caps aside. Finely chop about 1/2 the mushroom stems. (Use the surplus in another recipe or freeze for later use.)
Mix cream cheese, crab, chopped stems, lemon juice, Worcestershire sauce, basil, garlic powder, onions, and lemon pepper. Fill mushroom caps with the crab mixture and place in a large, lightly greased baking dish. Top with the grated Cheddar and Parmesan cheeses. (Recipe may be prepared to this point and refrigerated, covered, overnight.) Bake at 400°F for 15-20 minutes and serve warm.

Nutrition per Serving
Carbs: 1 g Fiber: 0 g **Net Carbs: 1 g** Protein: 3 g Fat: 4 g Calories: 55

Appetizers

Grilled Stuffed Mushrooms with Chorizo Stuffing

Servings: 24

24 large fresh white mushrooms (about 1 pound)
1/3 cup olive oil
5 ounces chorizo sausage (fully cooked), fine diced (about 1 cup)
1/4 cup chopped fresh parsley
2 large garlic cloves, finely chopped (about 2 teaspoons)

Prepare grill and vegetable grate or broiler and broiler pan. Remove mushroom stems. In a large bowl, combine mushroom caps and olive oil; toss to coat. In a small bowl, combine sausage, parsley and garlic. Fill mushroom cavities with sausage mixture. Place on vegetable grate or broiler pan. Grill or broil until mushrooms are tender and browned, 10 to 15 minutes.

Nutrition per Serving
Carbs: 1 g Fiber: 0 g **Net Carbs: 1 g** Protein: 5 g Fat: 16 g Calories: 171

Gregory Pryor C.E.C.

Appetizers

Stuffed Mushrooms with Feta Cheese
Servings: 24

24 large fresh white mushrooms (about 1 pound)
3 tablespoons olive oil, divided
1/3 cup chopped onion
2 teaspoons finely chopped garlic
1/3 cup pine nuts, toasted
1/2 teaspoon oregano leaves, crushed
1/8 teaspoon ground black pepper
4 ounces crumbled Feta (plain or flavored) or goat cheese, about 3/4 cup

Heat oven to 400ºF. Remove mushroom stems. Chop stems (makes about 1 cup); reserve. In a medium bowl, place caps; toss with 1 tablespoon of the oil. On a shallow baking pan, arrange mushroom caps, cavity side down; bake until tender, about 10 minutes. In a small skillet, over medium heat, heat remaining 2 tablespoons oil. Add onion, garlic and reserved mushroom stems; cook and stir until stems are tender and liquid evaporates, about 5 minutes. Stir in pine nuts, oregano and pepper. Transfer to a bowl; stir in Feta until mixture is well blended. Turn mushrooms over; stuff with cheese mixture. Bake until heated through, about 15 minutes; serve hot.

Nutrition per Serving
Carbs: 2 g Fiber: 1 g **Net Carbs: 1 g** Protein: 9 g Fat: 9 g Calories: 106

Appetizers

Smoked Salmon Cheese Ball
Servings: 18

A great way to serve this for a Low Carb treat, spread on fresh sliced cucumber rounds. Or slice the cucumbers about 1 1/2 inch thick and with a small melon scoop or a tablespoon, partially hollow out a circle in each slice and fill with cheese ball mixture. Therefore creating a cucumber canapé.

1 8-ounce package cream cheese at room temperature
1/4 cup grated Cheddar cheese
1/2 teaspoon horseradish
Dash Worcestershire sauce
1 teaspoon lemon juice
1 6 1/2-ounce can smoked salmon
1/2 cup ground pecans

Mix all ingredients together and roll into a ball. Roll in either chopped nuts or chives. Cover with plastic wrap and refrigerate until ready to use. (If smoked salmon is unavailable use canned salmon and 1/8 teaspoon of liquid smoke. Use more liquid smoke if you like a stronger flavor.)

Nutrition per Serving
Carbs: 2 g Fiber: 1 g **Net Carbs: 1 g** Protein: 10 g Fat: 21 g Calories: 232

Gregory Pryor C.E.C.

Appetizers

Saté of Pork
Servings: 8

Serve with peanut sauce. Consider using chicken, beef or lamb for this dish.

1 pound boneless pork loin
1/2 cup red wine vinegar
2 tablespoons olive oil
1 clove garlic, minced
1/4 teaspoon dried oregano, crushed
Cherry tomatoes (optional)

Partially freeze pork for 20-30 minutes; slice across the grain into 3 × 1 × 1/4-inch strips. Arrange pork in a shallow baking dish. For marinade, combine vinegar, olive oil, garlic and oregano; pour over pork. Cover and refrigerate 4 hours or overnight, turning pork occasionally.
Drain pork, reserving marinade. Thread pork on skewers. (If using wooden skewers, soak in water 20-30 minutes before using). Place skewers on grill about 4 inches over medium coals. Grill for 12-15 minutes, turning and brushing with marinade occasionally.
To Broil: Place skewers on rack in broiler pan. Broil about 5 inches from heat for 10-15 minutes, turning and brushing with marinade occasionally.

Nutrition per Serving
Carbs: 1 g Fiber: 0 g **Net Carbs: 1 g** Protein: 11 g Fat: 7 g Calories: 109

Sauces

Peanut Sauce
Servings: 18

Use only fresh ground unsweetened peanut butter. Most all health food stores have this item

1/3 cup peanut butter (natural), see above note
3 tablespoons rice wine vinegar
3 tablespoons water
1 tablespoon soy sauce
1 teaspoon sesame oil
1 clove garlic, finely chopped
1/2 tablespoon Splenda®
1/4 tablespoon red pepper flakes
2 tablespoons cilantro, finely chopped

In a medium bowl, mix peanut butter, vinegar, water, soy sauce, sesame oil, garlic, Splenda® and red pepper flakes until smooth Stir in cilantro. Add salt to taste

Nutrition per Serving
Carbs: 2 g Fiber: 0 g **Net Carbs: 2 g** Protein: 2 g Fat: 5 g Calories: 71

Gregory Pryor C.E.C.

Appetizers

Tuna Kebabs with Wasabi Mayonnaise
Servings: 10

To serve as an appetizer follow and serve as directed.
To serve as an entree' place four pieces tuna on four skewers and serve over fresh greens with a side vegetable.
As an entree' portion, cut the tuna into a bit larger pieces for 16 cubes.
To make cutting this tender fish easier, partially freeze the tuna 30-40 minutes before cutting.

1 cup mayonnaise
4 teaspoons soy sauce
1 1/2 teaspoons Splenda®
2 teaspoons fresh lemon juice
2 teaspoons Wasabi paste
1 12-16 ounce tuna steak, cut into twenty 1-inch cubes
10 8-inch bamboo skewers, soaked in water 30 minutes

In a bowl stir together mayonnaise, soy sauce, Splenda®, and lemon juice.
Transfer 2/3 cup soy mayonnaise to a small bowl and stir in Wasabi paste.
Stir tuna into remaining 1/3 cup soy mayonnaise.
Chill Wasabi mayonnaise, covered, at least 1-hour and up to 24.
Marinate tuna, covered and chilled, at least 1-hour and up to 24.
Prepare grill.
Thread 2 tuna cubes onto each skewer and grill on an oiled rack until just cooked through, 2 to 3 minutes on each side.
To Broil. Place skewers on broiler pan 4-6 inches below broiler, turning each till tuna is just cooked about 2 minutes a side.

Nutrition per Serving
Carbs: trace g Fiber: trace g **Net Carbs: trace g** Protein: 8 g Fat: 20 g Calories: 208

Appetizers

Asian Beef Skewers

Servings: 24

If using wooden skewers, soak in water 20-30 minutes before using

1 1/2 pounds flank steak
3/4 cup teriyaki sauce
6 tablespoons peanut oil
3 ounces fresh ginger root, finely chopped
1/3 cup garlic, minced
1 1/2 teaspoons red chili peppers, crushed

Prepare basting mixture by mixing teriyaki sauce, peanut oil, ginger, garlic and crushed red chili peppers. Cover and refrigerate.
Cut beef diagonally, against the grain, into 1/4 inch slices.
Thread each slice onto a bamboo skewer. Cover and chill.
For each serving: Brush 2 beef ribbons generously with basting mixture. Place skewers on grill about 4 inches over medium coals. Grill for 8-10 minutes, turning and brushing with marinade occasionally.
To Broil: Place skewers on rack in broiler pan. Broil about 5 inches from heat for 10-15 minutes, turning and brushing with marinade occasionally.

Nutrition per Serving
Carbs: 2 g Fiber: trace g **Net Carbs: 2 g** Protein: 6 g Fat: 6 g Calories: 93

Appetizers

Dijon Baby Back Ribs
Servings: 8

4 pounds baby back pork ribs
1 cup Mayonnaise
1/4 cup Dijon mustard
4 tablespoons Splenda®

If needed, cut ribs in lengths to fit in re-sealable plastic bag. Mix mayonnaise, mustard and Splenda®. Place ribs in bag and add the mayonnaise mixture; seal and marinate in refrigerator overnight. Discard used marinade and place ribs in a baking dish that has been sprayed with nonstick vegetable spray. Bake covered with foil in 300ºF oven for about 2 hours. Remove the foil the final 30 minutes or remove to a hot grill to finish cooking turning often so as not to burn.
Serving Ideas: Ribs may be cut into individual ribs before grilling and then served as appetizers or 'finger food'. Great for parties.

Nutrition per Serving
Carbs: trace g Fiber: trace g **Net Carbs: trace g** Protein: 25 g Fat: 57 g Calories: 605

Appetizers

Fish Cakes

Servings: 12

I use a bamboo Asian style steamer for this recipe. Lay some lettuce leaves on the bottom of the steamer if you use this approach. You can use any method that is within your kitchen to steam the fish. Also to add flavor, season your steaming liquid with a little white wine or Sake.

1 1/2 pound white fish fillets (with bones removed). Dolphin, Snapper, Sea bass etc.
1 teaspoon ginger paste
1 tablespoon lemon juice
1 medium green Chile (for a nice flavor and mild heat use jalapeno)
1 egg white
2 tablespoons cornstarch
1 tablespoon cilantro leaves, chopped
1 teaspoon cumin
1 teaspoon coriander powder
1 teaspoon garlic paste
1 medium onion, chopped finely
Salt, to taste
Clarified Butter for sautéing

Make diagonal slits on the fish and then steam it for ten minutes. Remove from heat and gently mash it with the remaining ingredients. Form mixture into walnut-sized balls and flatten slightly.

In a wide skillet heat oil on medium and when hot gently place the cakes in the skillet.

Let fry for two minutes and then turn over. Both sides must be golden-brown. Do not burn.

Serve hot. It is a good appetizer served with Remoulade sauce.

Nutrition per Serving
Carbs: 1 g Fiber: trace g **Net Carbs: 1 g** Protein: 8 g Fat: 2 g Calories: 56

Appetizers

Crab Cakes with Avocado Wasabi Mayonnaise

Servings: 4

1 pound lump crabmeat (Canned crabmeat – drained can be used)
3 tablespoons mayonnaise
1 teaspoon Worcestershire sauce
2 tablespoons fresh parsley
1 egg yolk
1 tablespoon Old Bay® seasoning
1 teaspoon lemon juice
1 tablespoon Dijon mustard
3 tablespoons fresh bread crumbs, 1 slice Low Carb bread dried or toasted
Avocado Wasabi Mayonnaise, see recipe

Gently pick through crabmeat to remove cartilage.
In mixing bowl gently combine all ingredients and portion into 2-ounce cakes.
Sauté in clarified butter until golden-brown on each side.
Serve with Avocado Wasabi Mayonnaise. Or Remoulade Sauce.

Nutrition per Serving
Carbs: 2 g Fiber: 1 g **Net Carbs: 1 g** Protein: 10 g Fat: 8 g Calories: 124

Appetizers

Avocado Wasabi Mayonnaise

1/2 cup mayonnaise
2 tablespoons Wasabi paste
1/2 avocado, peeled, seeded and puréed
3 tablespoons apple cider vinegar
Pinch salt
Pinch black pepper
Combine all ingredients well and chill.

Nutrition per Serving
Carbs: 3 g Fiber: 1 g **Net Carbs: 2 g** Protein: 1 g Fat: 8 g Calories: 105

Appetizers

Sweet and Sour Pork Meatballs

Who can resist sticking a tooth pick into a meatball and snacking?

1 pound lean ground pork
1/4 cup chopped onion
1 egg, slightly beaten
2 tablespoons soy sauce
1/8 teaspoon ground ginger
1 teaspoon vegetable oil
1 8-ounce can pineapple chunks
2 tablespoons soy sauce
1 tablespoon vinegar
1 tablespoon ThickenThin®
2 tablespoons Splenda®

In a large mixing bowl combine pork, onion, egg, 2 tablespoons soy sauce and ginger; shape into 1-inch balls. In a nonstick pan cook meatballs in hot oil until browned. Remove meatballs and drain, reserving drippings in skillet. Drain pineapple, reserving juice. In a 1-cup measure combine pineapple juice, 2 tablespoons soy sauce and vinegar. Add water to make 1 cup liquid. In mixing bowl combine ThickenThin® and Splenda®. Gradually stir in the pineapple juice mixture; mix well. Add juice mixture to pan drippings. Cook over medium heat until thickened and bubbly, stirring constantly. Stir in meatballs and the reserved pineapple. Cook for 4-5 minutes or until heated through.

Nutrition per Serving
Carbs: 1 g Fiber: trace g **Net Carbs: 1 g** Protein: 3 g Fat: 4 g Calories: 52

Basic Meatballs

Servings: 12 or 24 appetizer size

1 pound ground beef, 80% lean
1 egg, beaten
2 tablespoons onion, finely chopped
1/2 teaspoon salt

Place ground beef, egg, onion, and salt in bowl. Add specified ingredients to prepare Italian, Oriental or Swedish.

Nutrition per Serving
Carbs: trace g Fiber: trace g **Net Carbs: trace g** Protein: 7 g Fat: 10 g Calories: 123

Appetizers

Swedish Meatballs

Basic Meatball Mixture
1/8 teaspoon cardamom, ground
1 tablespoon vegetable oil
2 cups of brown sauce or beef broth
1/4 teaspoon dill weed
1 tablespoon ThickenThin®
1/2 cup sour cream

Combine ingredients of Basic Meatball Mixture with cardamom, mixing lightly but thoroughly. Shape mixture into 24 1 inch meatballs. Brown meatballs in hot oil in large skillet over medium heat. Pour off drippings. Add brown sauce or beef broth and dill weed to meatballs in skillet, stirring to combine. Bring to a boil; reduce heat. Add ThickenThin® cover tightly and simmer 20 minutes. Add sour cream just before service, mix well and serve in sauce.
Offer tooth picks for picking meatballs out of sauce.

Nutrition per Serving
Carbs: trace g Fiber: trace g **Net Carbs: trace g** Protein: trace g Fat: 2 g Calories: 15

Appetizers

Canadian-Bacon and Eggplant Roll-Ups

Servings: 10

10 slices Canadian bacon, about 1/8-inch thick (about 10 oz.)
1 large eggplant, about 1 1/2 pounds
3 tablespoons vegetable oil
2 tablespoons ThickenThin®
1 1/2 heavy cream
Dash ground pepper
Dash nutmeg
1 cup part-skim Ricotta cheese
2 tablespoons chopped parsley
2 tablespoons grated Parmesan cheese

Wash eggplant; pare if desired; cut off stem and blossom end. Cut lengthwise into 10 thin slices. Brush slices lightly with oil and sauté a few at a time in a 10-inch fry pan until tender. Set aside.

Measure 1 tablespoon of oil into fry pan; stir in ThickenThin®, add cream; cook and stir until mixture simmers and thickens. Take care not to boil this mixture over.

Season with pepper and nutmeg. Combine Ricotta cheese and parsley. Lay one slice of bacon on each eggplant slice.

Lap one small eggplant slice over a larger slice.

Spoon a rounded tablespoon of cheese over eggplant and bacon. Roll around cheese and place seam-side-down.

In an 11 × 7-inch baking dish. Pour sauce over eggplant roll-ups. Sprinkle with cheese. Bake in a 375°F oven for 30 minutes or until heated through.

Nutrition per Serving
Carbs: 2 g Fiber: 1 g **Net Carbs: 1 g** Protein: 11 g Fat: 10 g Calories: 158

As you can see from these ideas and recipes, with a little imagination and/or a change here or there you can expand you appetizer forte into an endless list of variations for whatever your situation calls for. Now speaking of imagination, remember earlier I said with a little experimenting and imagination you can even make Sushi rolls? Well, you can. I will outline just how to do that for you. All of us familiar with any Sushi roll know the one element to making the roll Low Carb is to replace the sweet rice. Ok so first let's look at the typical products you'll need to perform this task. Oh, and won't your Low Carb friends be envious when you tell them you had a California roll last night. Ok, typically the simplest thing to do if you're truly a lover of this is to get yourself a basic Sushi roll kit, consisting of a rolling matte, Wasabi, Nori or seaweed and in some cases a small jar of pickled ginger. I have seen several examples of these in local seafood stores, as well as any Asian market or specialty store. Once you have the essentials, the next step is to get the filling products. For this example we will use an English cucumber, avocado, crabmeat or imitation crabsticks, cream cheese and a sprinkle of sesame seeds (*optional*). Ok now once you have all this assembled, here is the trick to creating your Low Carb sweet rice. Oh, and before you go any further, take notice in takes practice to perfect the proper Sushi roll. Don't be disappointed if you find yourself making 4 or 5 before you get the knack.

So here we go. The rice in this case is cauliflower. Yes, that's right cauliflower. Because of its somewhat neutral taste and texture we can create a mock sweet sticky rice type replacement. So take half a head of cauliflower, remove only the floret's and trim away as much of the stalk as possible. Now take the floret's and with a box grater, using the medium holes, grate the cauliflower so it resembles rice. Once grated cook this for a few short minutes in boiling unsalted water. You will have to experiment with the time, but be certain to test the cauliflower and do not overcook. You will want it cooked just to the point of al dente. You will want the cauliflower to have a slight resistance when bitten. Immediately drain and rinse under cold water in a fine mess strainer to stop the cooking and set aside. Let this drain well. Now we have to make the "*dressing*". When normal Sushi rice is prepared it is dressed with a sugar and rice wine vinegar dressing. The difference here that is most noticeable is, when Sushi rice is cooked, the starch is what makes the rice sticky and pliable. So our next obstacle is to create both the sweetness and the mild stickiness we would expect from the actual rice. So we make our dressing:

Take 1/2 cup of rice wine vinegar and to this whisk in 1 tablespoon of Splenda®. Place the cauliflower in a large bowl and sprinkle lightly with the dressing. Being careful not to add so much dressing that it pools in the bowl. Mix gently but well. Now, to create the sticky part of our replica rice. Once the cauliflower is evenly coated with the dressing, sprinkle, a little, a time enough ThickenThin® to bring the cauliflower together. Allow to sit at intervals as needed for the ThickenThin® to tighten the cauliflower. Once this step is completed, you're ready to move on to the basic assembly of the Sushi roll. Begin with first peeling the cucumber and slicing this in long approx 3/8" inch thick slices. Then again lengthwise slice 3/8" slices. Finally trim these squares the same length as the Nori is wide. Now cut the avocado in half down to the pit, separate the avocado and remove the pit. Cut these halves into quarters and peel. Continue to make thin slices of the quarters and set aside. Slice several 1/4" slices of the cream cheese and set aside:

Hopefully the Sushi kit you bought you will have an illustration of how to roll a Sushi roll. Lay out your rolling matte. If the matte you bought is not covered in plastic wrap do so now. Once you have the matte ready and laid out in front of you, take one sheet of Nori and cut in half (or you can use the whole sheet). Just experiment till you have the size that's easiest for you to work with. Lay the Nori on the matte and spread a thin layer of the cauliflower over the Nori. Make certain to keep this even without any voids on the surface, leaving approx a 1/4" of bare Nori at the bottom edge away from you. Now you can place your fillings onto the roll. First sprinkle a light coating of sesame seeds over the cauliflower. Next lay an even line of crabmeat or a stick of imitation if you choose, approx

1/2" from the edge closes to you, followed with two slices of avocado going from side to side. Finish with a slice of cream cheese:

Ok, now the tricky part. Holding your fingers over the roll, use your fingers and thumbs to grasp the matte and lift the edge closest to you up and over the filling. Making a small tube, so to speak. Once you're at this point simply in one motion roll the matte and Sushi roll as you would a jelly roll. Assuming all went well, at this point you should have a nicely rolled Sushi roll. Now lay your matte over the roll and with a gentle, yet firm pressure shape the roll evenly into a cylinder. Finally, with a sharp knife, cut the roll in half at the center point. What I do at this point is lay each half next to each other. Now cut each of these halves into 4 pieces, for a total of eight pieces. Now there you have it, Low Carb Sushi Roll. Serve with soy sauce and Wasabi. Once you master this technique you can then make any type of Sushi roll you desire. Once you learn to experiment and *"think outside the box"*, converting most dishes or recipes will become a rewarding experience in your kitchen.

DIPS AND SALSA

In the typical high carb world we would normally associate dips and salsa's as not being something included in our Low Carb Lifestyle. Think about that, wouldn't you agree that what comes to mind are examples such as; Chips and Dip, or how about that refried bean and tortilla chips concoction. Again these examples come to mind simply because that is the normal association we have with dips and salsas. This just isn't the case in the Low Carb Lifestyle. Dips and Salsa's have every bit as much a place in our lifestyle as they did before in the typical high carb cuisines we grew up with. One of the recipes I have offered in this book is one I call root chips. These wonderful alternatives to typical chips are matched enjoyably with any of the following recipes. Another wonderful and creative use of many of these salsas is as an accompaniment to many of the Beef, Poultry and Fish entrée's. Here is a great example. Grilled Swordfish with roasted garlic salsa. The combinations are endless once you begin paring different flavors. Another wonderful use of Low Carb dips and salsa is with the fresh array of crudités' we have offered in this book. Dips can be as simple as a combination of sour cream and mayonnaise with some Creole spice added to taste, or even seafood dip. What I suggest here is that you experiment with these various dips and salsas, not only in the traditional use of chips and dip, but as accompaniments to other entrée dishes.

Gregory Pryor C.E.C.

Appetizers & Snacks

Root Chips
Servings: 6 - 8

These mock potato chips taste better and are easy to make.
To ensure a perfect slice, I use a slicer or a mandolin. If you own a mandolin you can cut these to resemble wavy chips or ruffles. For dipping purposes this will make the chip stronger. But the key is to slice each slice as thin as possible, and be consistent.

4 ounces rutabaga, thinly sliced
4 ounces jicama, thinly sliced
4 ounces celery root, thinly sliced
2 cups vegetable oil

With a sharp knife or vegetable peeler, peel then slice each vegetable in thin 1/8 inch slices.
Place the sliced vegetables in a bowl of cold water to prevent discoloration.
Heat in a deep fryer or heavy pot with 2 inches of oil to 350 degree's.
Drain and pat dry the vegetables. Fry each type separate and fry till golden-brown.
The time will vary with each vegetable. Continue and drain on a paper towel.
Season to taste with salt and serve warm. Or keep in an airtight container for up to 3 days.

Nutrition per Serving
Carbs: 4 g Fiber: 2 g **Net Carbs: 2 g** Protein: trace g Fat: 73 g Calories: 659

Dips/Salsa

Black Olive Aioli Dip

1 cup mayonnaise
1/4 cup black olives, ground
2 cloves garlic, minced
2 teaspoons lemon juice
1/4 cup parsley, chopped
Salt and pepper, to taste

Combine mayonnaise, black olives, garlic, lemon juice and chopped parsley. Add salt and pepper to taste.

Nutrition per Serving
Carbs: trace g Fiber: trace g **Net Carbs: trace g** Protein: trace g Fat: 16 g Calories: 136

Dips/Salsa

Chimichurri Sauce
Servings: 6

Here is another of those sauces that one can alter in many ways to adapt flavors or needs. I enjoy this as a spicy sauce for fish. Replace one fresh jalapeno pepper with either a half or whole depending on heat, chipotle pepper finely chopped and 1/2 teaspoon of the adobo sauce. This makes a wonderful zesty red sauce. Be certain to use caution when using these fiery peppers.

1 cup parsley, flat leaf
6 cloves garlic, peeled
2 jalapeno peppers, seeded
5 tablespoons extra virgin olive oil
3 tablespoons red wine vinegar
1 teaspoon kosher salt
1/4 teaspoon Old Bay® Seafood seasoning

In a food processor, combine parsley, garlic and jalapenos; process until a chunky paste forms. Drizzle in oil while pulsing processor, stir in vinegar, and add Old Bay® seasoning, season to taste with salt.

Nutrition per Serving
Carbs: 2 g Fiber: 1 g **Net Carbs: 1 g** Protein: 1 g Fat: 11 g Calories: 110

Dips/Salsa

Crab Dip
Servings: 6

Here is a great dip that you can alter to match your needs or taste. Add any combination of chopped celery jalapeno peppers, Chipotle peppers or another other added flavors that match your needs or desires.
To clean crabmeat; spread crabmeat evenly on a cookie sheet. Place in a 300 degree oven for about 10 minutes.
Remove from the oven and let cool to the touch. Look for any white or cream colored bits, these are bits of shell.
Do not use imitation crabmeat, this is full of carbs.

1/4 cup mayonnaise
1/4 cup sour cream
1 teaspoon Old Bay® Seafood seasoning
1 teaspoon lemon juice, fresh
6 ounces crabmeat, see note
2 green onions, finely chopped
2 tablespoons red bell pepper, finely chopped
1 dash Worcestershire sauce

In a medium bowl, mix mayonnaise, sour cream, seasoning and lemon juice until smooth. Add crab, green onions and pepper; stir until ingredients are well combined. Stir in a dash of Worcester sauce. Season to taste with salt and pepper.

Nutrition per Serving
Carbs: 6 g Fiber: 1 g **Net Carbs: 5 g** Protein: 38 g Fat: 61 g Calories: 702

Dips/Salsa

Halibut Dip

Servings: 8

Poached Halibut: Cover halibut, thawed if necessary, with boiling, salted water. Add 2 slices onion, 2 slices lemon, 4 sprigs parsley and several peppercorns. Simmer, covered, allowing 10 minutes per inch of thickness measured at its thickest part or until halibut flakes easily when tested with a fork. You can substitute any firm white fish such as, Sea bass, Grouper etc. Being certain you choose a mild white fish. This is another wonderful filling for stuffed mushrooms, simply mound mushroom caps and bake till golden-brown.

12 ounces poached halibut see notes
1 8-ounce package cream cheese, softened
2 tablespoons lemon juice
2 teaspoons grated onion
1 teaspoon Worcestershire sauce
1/2 teaspoon salt
1/4 teaspoon garlic salt
1/4 teaspoon dill weed, crushed
Dash bottled hot pepper sauce
Parsley sprigs

Flake halibut; combine with cream cheese. Add lemon juice, onion and seasonings. Blend thoroughly in food processor or electric mixer.
Press mixture into bowl or mold lined with plastic wrap. Refrigerate several hours or overnight. Unmold onto serving platter; garnish with parsley. Serve with crisp fresh vegetables.

Nutrition per Serving
Carbs: 1 g Fiber: 0 g **Net Carbs: 1 g** Protein: 11 g Fat: 11 g Calories: 147

Gregory Pryor C.E.C.

Dips/Salsa

Pico de Gallo Relish
Servings: 8

I prefer pebbly skinned Haas avocados: the flavor is richer and the texture much creamier.
I serve this as a condiment to grilled pork and fish.

1 avocado, chopped
1 tomato, chopped
3 onions, chopped
1 jalapeno, finely chopped
3 tablespoons cilantro, finely chopped
1 tablespoon lemon juice
1 tablespoon canola oil
Salt and pepper, to taste

In a small bowl, combine all ingredients. Add salt and pepper to taste. Refrigerate 4 hours to blend flavors.

Nutrition per Serving
Carbs: 7 g Fiber: 2 g **Net Carbs: 5 g** Protein: 1 g Fat: 6 g Calories: 77

Dips/Salsa

Spinach Dip
Servings: 12

1 10-ounce package frozen chopped spinach, thawed
1 cup mayonnaise
1 cup sour cream
1/2 cup chopped fresh parsley
1/2 cup chopped green onions
1 clove garlic, minced
Salt and pepper

Drain spinach and squeeze dry. In a bowl, combine dip ingredients; season with salt and pepper; Chill 8 hours or overnight. Adjust seasoning before serving.
Yield: 3 cups

Nutrition per Serving
Carbs: 1 g Fiber: 0 g **Net Carbs: 1 g** Protein: 1g Fat: 10 g Calories: 90

Dips/Salsa

Clam and Olive Dip

Servings: 8

1 can black olives, drained and chopped
1 can clams, minced and drained
1 cup sour cream
1 teaspoon salt
1 teaspoon garlic powder
1 teaspoon dried parsley
1/2 teaspoon cayenne pepper, or to taste

Mix together all the ingredients, stir, and chill for 2 hours before serving.

Nutrition per Serving
Carbs: 2 g Fiber: trace g **Net Carbs: 2 g** Protein: 6 g Fat: 6 g Calories: 93

Dips/Salsa

Tomatillo Salsa
Servings: 10

This wonderful fruit is often referred to as a Mexican green tomato. The flavor of these lends itself well for salsa and dip. For an even greater robust flavor, roast the tomatillos before use in salsa or dip. This is another one of those salsa's that goes wonderful with roasted pork, grilled fish, and grilled southwestern steaks.

6 tomatillos, whole, peeled and chopped
1 tomatoes, whole, chopped
1/2 red onion, diced
1 jalapeno pepper, chopped
1 tablespoon cilantro
1 teaspoon oregano
1 teaspoon ground cumin
1 teaspoon salt
1 teaspoon ground black pepper
1 lime

Combine the tomatillos, tomatoes, red onion, garlic, jalapeno, cilantro, oregano, cumin, and salt in the bowl of a food processor. Juice the lime into the mixture. Pulse until the mixture is well-blended and all the ingredients are roughly chopped.

Nutrition per Serving
Carbs: 3 g Fiber: 1 g **Net Carbs: 2 g** Protein: 1 g Fat: trace g Calories: 17

Dips/Salsa

Bubbly Hot Cheese Dip
Servings: 8

You can substitute any hard cheese to create a dip for your occasion. Serve with root chips.

8 ounces cheddar cheese, shredded
1 cup mayonnaise
1/2 medium onion, shredded
1 tablespoon horseradish

Lightly butter a 6-inch soufflé dish or an 8-inch baking dish. Combine ingredients. Pour into dish. Bake at 375 degrees for 15 minutes until bubbly and brown around the edges.

Nutrition per Serving
Carbs: 1 g Fiber: 0 g **Net Carbs: 1 g** Protein: 7 g Fat: 33 g Calories: 315

Dips/Salsa

Crudité Dip 1
Servings: 12

This is a great dip to serve with crisp fresh vegetables.

1/2 cup mayonnaise
1/2 cup sour cream
2 teaspoons chili sauce
2 teaspoons chives, chopped
2 teaspoons onion, grated
1/2 teaspoon curry powder

In a large bowl, combine all the ingredients, mix well and chill before service.

Nutrition per Serving
Carbs: 1 g Fiber: 0 g **Net Carbs: 1 g** Protein: trace g Fat: 10 g Calories: 87

Gregory Pryor C.E.C.

Dips/Salsa

Crudité Dip 2
Servings: 24

1 cup mayonnaise
1 cup sour cream
4 ounces cream cheese, softened
1 tablespoon lemon juice
1 dash Tabasco sauce
1 tablespoon dried chives, or fresh
1 tablespoon garlic powder
2 tablespoons dill weed
1 tablespoon paprika

In a large bowl, combine mayonnaise, sour cream and cream cheese. Mix well till cream cheese is smooth. You can use a kitchen aide with a paddle to make mixing much easier.
Add remaining ingredients and blend well. Allow mixture to chill 4-24 hours before service.

Nutrition per Serving
Carbs: 1 g Fiber: 0 g **Net Carbs: 1 g** Protein: 1 g Fat: 11 g Calories: 106

Dips/Salsa

Blue Cheese Dip
Servings: 8

1/2 cup mayonnaise
1/2 cup sour cream
3 ounces crumbled bleu cheese
1 tablespoon buttermilk
Salt and white pepper, to taste

In a large bowl, combine first 3 ingredients. Thin to desired consistency with buttermilk, season to taste with salt and pepper.

Nutrition per Serving
Carbs: 1 g Fiber: 0 g **Net Carbs: 1 g** Protein: 4 g Fat: 24 g Calories: 224

Dips/Salsa

Hot Artichoke Dip
Servings: 12

I like to serve this with fresh vegetables and root chips.

1 can artichoke hearts, drained and chopped
1 cup sour cream
1 cup parmesan cheese, grated
1 clove garlic, minced
1 teaspoon salt
2 teaspoons paprika

Mix all ingredients, pour into a buttered 8-inch baking dish, sprinkle with paprika and bake at 350 for 30 minutes or until bubbly.

Nutrition per Serving
Carbs: 2 g Fiber: 1 g **Net Carbs: 1 g** Protein: 4 g Fat: 6 g Calories: 76

It is my wish, after reading and using these dip and salsa recipes you're able to conclude that we have many choices in the Low Carb Lifestyle. From the examples I have provided I also feel certain that you can now feel confident in knowing that this lifestyle is far from boring.

Now that we have taken some time and explored the appetizers, dips and salsas, let's get serious about cooking. Now we will look at those wonderful, classical stocks and sauces. The variations are nearly endless as to what you will be able to create to add flavors to your dishes, as well as create simply wonderful rich, satisfying soups.

STOCKS AND SAUCES

When I was in Culinary School, by far one of my favorite subjects was stocks and sauces. I was always considered by my instructors and fellow students to be a natural. Long after Culinary School as I was working my way through the various levels to becoming an Executive Chef my stock and sauce skills were always well appreciated in every establishment I worked in. Having boasted a bit now let's look at the principles of stock and sauce making. With but few exceptions, the principles of Classical and Low Carb are almost identical. The only significant difference is that we will omit or limit the use of roux in our Low Carb sauces. However, we will occasionally use a roux when practical and, as you will see, the small amount we will use adds so little net carbs that we are still able to use the typical and classical roux, when needed.

Now to understand the difference of these two critical and useful items, let me give you a concise outline of stocks and sauces. Of course both of these date back perhaps centuries to the evolution of classical cooking. Even still little other than the modernization of cookware and product has changed. The principles remain the same.

Stock is a flavored liquid. A good stock is the basis for a great soup, sauce or braised dish. The French refer to a stock as stock fond (base), as stocks are the basis for many classical and modern dishes.

Sauce is a thickened liquid used to flavor and improve other foods. A quality sauce adds flavor, moisture, richness and visual appeal. A sauce should compliment food, it should never disguise it. Sauces, once made properly should be used sparingly. The rich intense flavors should enhance not hinder the food they are served with. Do not allow the main item to "*swim*" in a sauce. Sauces can be hot or cold, sweet or savory, smooth or chunky. Over the years many people I have met, both professional and home cooks, have suggested that making these stocks and sauces can be intimidating. The truth is that the procedures are simple and with a little practice and time, you will be just at ease making these as you are with any other common cooking technique.

What we will review here are five basic stocks from which hundreds of sauces and soup bases can be prepared.

White stock is fairly clear made by simmering chicken, veal or beef bones in water with vegetables and seasonings. I cannot emphasis strongly enough the importance of a controlled slow simmer. Rapid cooking of a stock will result in a cloudy unattractive stock.

Brown Stock is rich dark stock made by simmering chicken, veal or beef bones and vegetables that have been cooked or (*caramelized*) before being simmered in water.

Fish Stock and **Fumet** are made by slowly cooking fish bones or crustacean shells and vegetables without browning them, then adding cold water and seasonings and simmering for a short period of time. For a fumet, wine and lemon juices are added. Both are strongly flavored, fairly clear stocks.

Court Bouillon is most commonly used to poach fish and vegetables. It is made by simmering vegetables and seasonings in water with an added acid such as vinegar or wine.

The ingredients of any stock are essentially the same, bones, vegetables (*mirepoix*), seasonings and water. Bones are the most important part or ingredient to producing a quality stock. The bones add flavor color, and richness. Because the way that most cuts of beef are now sent to the butcher and supermarkets, you may have to ask the butcher to order you the beef and veal bones. Alternately you may ask him or her to save them for you.

In the commercial kitchen these days we have to order the bones we need to make these stocks. Most any butcher shop will be happy to sell you bones for stock making. In fact, when you tell the butcher what these bones will be used for, he will know what types of bones you need and should offer to cut them into 3 to 4 inch pieces. Since different bones release their flavors at different rates, stocks made of veal and beef bones will require a simmering time of 6-8 hours, while a stock made of chicken bones needs 4-5 hours simmering time. No matter what bones you are using chicken or veal and beef, the best bones for making a stock come from the necks and backs of the animal. To create a full bodied and rich brown stock it is crucial that you have good quality veal and beef bones from as young an animal as possible. These bones contain a higher concentration of cartilage than do the bones of older animals. This cartilage is high in collagen, which is the basis for the gelatin richness and body of a good stock, and the magic to creating a thick rich reduction. It is for this reason that we can make those thick sauces from homemade stocks that need little if any roux. This is something we just cannot do using canned broth.

Ok, I know what you're thinking, this sounds like a lot of work. Actually in truth it is not if you're prepared and organized in your task. A little later I will explain how you can make many of these stock-based sauces ala' minute, or in the pan. More on that later. However the effort this procedure takes is far more rewarding in the finished product and what all we can do with these stocks makes it worth the time. Finally these stocks freeze well. It is a simple task to package the cooled stock in small airtight plastic containers and stack them in your freezer to use as needed. For chicken stock the same necks and backs are the best choices for this stock. When getting bones for a fish stock, avoid any of the fatty fishes such as salmon, tuna and swordfish. Most fishmongers or fish markets are more than happy to give you these bones and carcasses. Before using these bones, always take them home and clean any loose scales, blood spots or other nonbone particles by running them under cold water and scraping them if necessary. Using a heavy kitchen knife or cleaver chop or cut the carcasses into smaller pieces before cooking.

A nother essential ingredient in stock making is the vegetables or **mirepoix**. Traditionally the vegetables used are carrots, onion and celery. Although many Chefs differ on the ratio of these vegetables, classically the ratio is 50% onion, 25% carrot and 25% celery. For our Low Carb stocks we will use this ratio as the carrots would contribute a few extra net carbs should we increase this ratio. Actually when we make our chicken and fish stock we can eliminate the carrots completely and replace them with leeks. These vegetables do not need to be peeled, simply cleaned before chopping or cutting. In fact, the onion skins contain a lot of flavor when cooked: Seasonings when making a stock are peppercorns, bay leaves, thyme and or parsley stems and garlic (optionally). I will tell you I never use garlic in stock making for several reasons. One is more and more people have sensitivity to garlic. Second, many of the sauces we would make would not benefit from the garlic. So I simply make and add a **bouquet garni**, that consist of whole peppercorns 10-12, 2 bay leaves and 6-8 parsley stems. Never add salt to a stock. As the stock cooks and reduces the salt will intensify and can overpower the stock. We always season the stock or sauce to taste during the final cooking stage. Finally, both during and after the stock is cooled, we want to remove as much fat as the stock may produce. Now here are the principles of stock making:

Start the stock in cold water

Simmer the stock gently

Skim the stock often

Cool the stock quickly

Store the stock properly

Degrease the stock

Now as promised before, let's talk for a minute about making a sauce or stock based sauce ala' minute, or in the pan. Sometimes when preparing a dish for just one or two people it is just not always practical to make a stock before making the dish. Another reason for making a sauce in the pan simply is ease and speed. This method requires very little effort or time, but doesn't produce the same robust rich flavor and texture as a long slow simmered stock. Fortunately now that we have ThickenThin® we can make these pan sauces without the high carb addition of roux. To make this sauce you still need some bones and mirepoix. However usually these bones are a result of the meat item we are using for the recipe. For example you can buy whole on the bone chicken breast and debone them yourself, or ask the butcher to do so and save the bones for you to take home. To make you're in the pan sauce, once you have sautéed the meat item, remove and hold the item in a warm place, taking care not to overcook. You can always return the item to the sauce to finish cooking or to heat through. In the same sauté pan add the bones and a handful of mirepoix to the pan. Cook till everything is well caramelized. Finally deglaze the pan with the bones and mirepoix in it with either canned broth beef or chicken depending on the sauce. If you do not have any canned broth you can use a little white or red wine and water. Let this simmer and reduce by 1/3. Strain the sauce, return to the pan, swirl in some cold butter, thicken with ThickenThin® if needed and serve with the meat you have holding. Although I honestly prefer to have fresh stock available to complete the sauce used in the many recipes in this book. Most all the sauces we will make that go with a recipe are pan sauces but usually finished using slow cooked stocks. You will see as you follow the recipes that most sauces are simply an addition of a few items to the sauté pan and finished by adding the stock and reduce the final sauce. Now as we look at the following stock and sauce recipes you will see how we use various additives to a base stock or sauce to create countless smaller sauces from the stock and or mother sauces. Not all sauces are made from slow cooked stocks, although the greatest numbers of sauces do originate from these stocks. Some of the sauces we will be using are rich butter sauces, different from stock based sauces.

Many of the recipes in this book will call for stock, especially soups, sauces and braised items. Substituting canned broth will work, but again, the loss of texture and rich flavor is very noticeable. So please, to fulfill that promise of rich flavorful recipes I made earlier, I strongly urge you to make these fresh stocks. Now I will share a shortcut secret with you. Although the following product is somewhat expensive, the quality is unsurpassed and naturally Low in Carbs. These products are stock bases that can be used to make perfect stocks and sauces. Please visit my web site www.lowcarbchef.net for further information on these products.

Stocks

Basic Brown Stock

One of the most popular stocks used by professional chefs and more home cooks is a basic brown stock. The reason for its popularity? It is the foundation for making several sauces including brown sauce, Demi-glace, and pan sauces. When reduced to thick syrup it is called Glace de Viande. As well as being critical in sauce making, Brown Stock and Glace de Viande are often used as a base for soups and braises and give any dish added flavor and color.
It is not difficult to make but does take a lot of time and equipment to make basic brown stock and if you want to prepare a Glace de Viande, it takes even longer, but the reward is well worth the effort.
Once finished this stock freezes well.

4 pounds veal bones, cut 2-4 inch length
3 pounds beef marrow bones, cut 2-4 inch length
4 ounces tomato paste
2 cups onion, chopped
1 cup carrot, chopped
1 cup celery, chopped
2 cups dry red wine
BOUQUET GARNI
8 quarts water

Preheat the oven to 450 degrees F. Place the bones in a roasting pan and roast for 1-hour.
Remove the bones from the oven and brush with the tomato paste.
Combine the onions, carrots, and celery together. Lay the vegetables over the bones and return to the oven. Roast for 30 minutes. Remove from the oven and drain off any fat.
Place the roasting pan on the stove and deglaze the pan with the red wine, using a wooden spoon, scraping the bottom of the pan for browned particles. Put everything into a large stockpot. Add the bouquet garni. Add the water. Bring the liquid up to a boil and reduce to a simmer. Simmer the stock for 6 to 8 hours, skimming regularly.
Remove from the heat and strain through a China cap or tightly meshed strainer lined with cheesecloth.

Nutrition per Serving 2 oz.
Carbs: 2 g Fiber: 1 g **Net Carbs: 1 g** Protein: trace g Fat: trace g Calories: 23

Stocks

Chicken Stock

This is another essential stock for sauces, soups and all around cooking use. If you have a local butcher shop you should be able to buy necks and backs for a very affordable price. If not, most supermarkets sell these at a slightly higher cost. For the basic simmered stock version trim away as much of the fat from the chicken as possible.

To make a darker richer stock, oven roast the bones and parts till a dark brown, then continue as a simmered stock as directed in this recipe. The best aspect of homemade stock is the wonderful body and flavor as opposed to canned broth. A rich chicken stock when chilled should be a thick gelatin type texture which you do not get using canned broth. This gelatin texture is what improves the soups and sauces we will make using chicken stock.

I especially prefer the roasted version for sauces, but prefer the simmered version, which is clear for soups.

5 pounds chicken backs and necks
1 large onion, quartered
1 large leek, cut into 2" pieces
4 stalks celery, cut into 2" pieces
Bouquet Garni

Place all the ingredients in an 8-quart stockpot and cover with cold water. Bring to a boil over high heat. As the stock approaches a boil, remove any impurities that rise to the top by skimming with a ladle. Reduce the heat and simmer the stock uncovered for 5 to 6 hours, continuing to skim impurities while the stock cooks.

Taste after 3 hours for the strength of stock you want. Remove from the heat and let the sock sit for 10 to 15 minutes, then ladle through a fine strainer.

Once strained, remove the fat from the stock by skimming with a ladle.

Another way to defat the sock is to place the cooled stock in the refrigerator overnight. The fat will set on the top and can be easily spooned off. However if your going to store the stock fresh and not frozen, leave this fat cover on the stock, it will protect the stock during storage.

The stock will keep for about 1 week in the refrigerator, or freeze in plastic airtight containers of the size you will use on an as needed basis, like 1 cup size.

Nutrition per Serving 2 oz
Carbs: 1 g Fiber: 0 g **Net Carbs: 1 g** Protein: 2 g Fat: 2 g Calories: 73

Stocks

Fish Stock

Fish stock is also known as fish fumet. Make sure the fish bones you use are from lean fish and not fatty fish (avoid salmon, tuna or trout bones, for instance).
Most any seafood market will give these bones away. It is best to call ahead of time and ask them to save you the bones you need. They will know when you tell them you're making fish stock just what you need.

6 pounds fish bones
2 tablespoons butter, unsalted
1/2 large onion, diced
3 stalks celery, diced
1 large leek, chopped
6 quarts cold water
1 cup dry white wine
Bouquet Garni

Melt the butter in the bottom of a large stockpot. Add the mirepoix (onions, celery and leek), and place the bones on top.
Sweat the mirepoix and bones stirring over low heat for about 5 minutes, until the bones turn opaque and release some juices.
Add the wine, bring to a simmer. Add the Bouquet Garni and water.
Bring to a simmer, skim any scum that forms, and continue to simmer for 45 minutes. Strain through a fine mess strainer layered with cheesecloth. Cool the stock immediately in an ice water bath, transfer to a container and refrigerate. Skim off any fat that rises to the top.
Store in a covered container for up to 1 week in the refrigerator, or freeze in airtight plastic containers in sizes that will best suit your needs. Thaw as needed.

Nutrition per Serving
Carbs: 1 g Fiber: trace g **Net Carbs: 1 g** Protein: trace g Fat: 1 g Calories: 18

Gregory Pryor C.E.C.

Sauces

Tomato Sauce

Servings: 4

This is a simple Low Carb version of tomato or a marinara type sauce. Many times when I need or want tomato sauce for a dish, I simply use Natural no sugar added canned diced tomatoes, heated in a sauté pan; add some fresh basil and season to taste. I enjoy this every bit as much as a long cooked tomato sauce.

1 tablespoon olive oil
2 teaspoons chopped fresh thyme
1/2 cup basil, fresh, torn
1 pound ripe tomatoes, peeled, seeded and diced
Salt and pepper

Heat the olive oil in a pan.
Stir in all the remaining ingredients.
Simmer gently for 15 minutes.
Purée or pulse in a blender until either chunky or smooth.
Return to the pan and keep warm.

Nutrition per Serving 4 oz
Carbs: 5 g Fiber: 1 g **Net Carbs: 4 g** Protein: 1 g Fat: 4 g Calories: 53

Sauces

Hollandaise Sauce

Servings: 4

Sauce should have the texture of mayonnaise

1 teaspoon shallot, finely chopped
1/4 cup white wine vinegar
1 tablespoon lemon juice
2 egg yolks, plus 1 tablespoon water
4 ounces clarified butter
Salt, to taste
White pepper, to taste
Cayenne pepper, to taste

In a double boiler (or heatproof bowl set over, but not touching, a saucepot of simmering water), combine shallot, vinegar and lemon juice. Cook 5 minutes, until most of the vinegar has evaporated. Whisk in egg yolk mixture. Whisk continuously until egg yolks have thickened, about 5 minutes. Whisk in butter gradually, in a slow drip/stream, until incorporated. Remove from heat. Season to taste with salt and pepper. Add a pinch of cayenne pepper, stir to blend.

Nutrition per Serving
Carbs: 1 g Fiber: 0 g **Net Carbs: 1 g** Protein: 2 g Fat: 31 g Calories: 282

Gregory Pryor C.E.C.

Sauces

Béarnaise Sauce
Servings: 4

1 shallot, finely chopped
1 1/2 teaspoons tarragon, fresh finely chopped
1 teaspoon chervil, fresh finely chopped
1/4 cup white wine vinegar
1 tablespoon lemon juice
2 egg yolks, plus 1 tablespoon water
4 ounces clarified butter
Salt, to taste
White pepper, to taste

In a double boiler or heatproof bowl set over, but not touching, a saucepot of simmering water, combine shallot, tarragon, chervil, vinegar and lemon juice. Cook, until most of the vinegar has evaporated. Whisk in egg yolk mixture. Whisk continuously until egg yolks have thickened, about 5 minutes. Whisk in butter gradually, in a slow drip/stream, until incorporated. Remove from heat. Season to taste with salt and pepper.

Nutrition per Serving
Carbs: 2 g Fiber: 0 g **Net Carbs: 2 g** Protein: 2 g Fat: 31 g Calories: 285

Sauces

Cheese Sauce 1

This is a versatile cheese sauce. You can use most any real cheese, such as Cheddar, Provolone, Swiss, Montery Jack, etc. Use whatever flavor you wish to accomplish. Looking for a smoked cheese flavored sauce, remove the blue cheese and Jarlsberg and replace the same amount with smoked Gouda.
When making this sauce as a topping for steamed vegetables or for creamed spinach, sweat one fine chopped shallot and add to the warm cream.

1 cup heavy cream
1/2 cup blue cheese, crumbled
1/2 cup Jarlsberg cheese, shredded
1/4 cup Parmesan cheese, grated
Pinch salt, to taste
Pinch black pepper, to taste

Heat cream in a large heavy saucepan over low heat. Do not boil.
Add blue cheese, stir until melted. Stir in Jarlsberg until melted. Add Parmesan and paprika.
Continue cooking, stirring, until sauce is smooth and hot. Season to taste with salt and pepper.

Nutrition per Serving
Carbs: 1 g Fiber: 0 g **Net Carbs: 1 g** Protein: 2 g Fat: 8 g Calories: 82

Gregory Pryor C.E.C.

Sauces

Cheese Sauce 2

This is another simple easy Low Carb Cheese sauce. I especially enjoy this version as the brie adds a creamy texture and just the right amount of "twang" to the sauce. I use this on a frequent basis as a thickener for creamed vegetables, especially creamed spinach. Brie has become so common and affordable these days it is a perfect choice for this sauce.

1 cup heavy cream
1/2 cup soft brie cheese, rind removed
1/2 cup Jarlsberg cheese, shredded
Pinch salt, to taste
Pinch black pepper, to taste

Heat cream in a large heavy saucepan over low heat. Do not boil.
Add brie, stir until melted. Stir in Jarlsberg until melted. Add paprika.
Continue cooking, stirring, until sauce is smooth and hot. Season to taste with salt and pepper.

Nutrition per Serving
Carbs: 1 g Fiber: 0 g **Net Carbs: 1 g** Protein: 2 g Fat: 8 g Calories: 82

Sauces

Choron Sauce
Servings: 4

1 shallot, finely chopped
1/4 cup white wine vinegar
1 tablespoon lemon juice
2 egg yolks, plus 1 tablespoon water
4 ounces clarified butter
1 tablespoon tomato paste
2 tablespoons heavy cream
Salt, to taste
White pepper, to taste
1 pinch cayenne pepper, to taste

In a double boiler or heatproof bowl set over, but not touching, a saucepot of simmering water, combine shallot, vinegar and lemon juice. Cook, until most of the vinegar has evaporated.

Whisk in egg yolk mixture. Whisk continuously until egg yolks have thickened, about 5 minutes. Whisk in butter gradually, in a slow drip/stream, until incorporated.

Add in the tomato sauce and cream, mix well.

Remove from heat. Season to taste with salt and pepper.

Nutrition per Serving
Carbs: 3 g Fiber: trace g **Net Carbs: 3 g** Protein: 2 g Fat: 34 g Calories: 312

Gregory Pryor C.E.C.

Sauces

Bordelaise Sauce
Servings: 4

The simple key to this sauce is the reduction. As the brown stock reduces it with thicken and intensify in flavor.

2 tablespoons clarified butter
1 whole shallot, minced
1 clove garlic, minced fine (optional)
1 cup brown stock
1/4 cup dry red wine
1 tablespoon cold butter

Melt the butter in a heavy skillet and sauté the shallot until transparent. Add garlic and sauté 1-minute, do not brown garlic. Add the brown stock and red wine and bring to a simmer and allow to reduce by 1/3 or until slightly thickened. Remove from the heat and add cold butter, swirl the pan to blend. Serve hot.

Nutrition per Serving
Carbs: 1 g Fiber: 0 g **Net Carbs: 1 g** Protein: trace g Fat: 9 g Calories: 95

Sauces

Mushroom Sauce

Servings: 4

The simple key to this sauce is the reduction. As the brown stock reduces it with thicken and intensify in flavor.
You choose any shape mushroom that pleases you, sliced, halved, or quartered.

2 tablespoons clarified butter
1 whole shallot, minced
1 clove garlic, minced fine (optional)
1/2 cup mushrooms
1 cup brown stock
1/4 cup dry red wine
1 tablespoon cold butter

Melt the butter in a heavy skillet and sauté the shallot until transparent.
Add garlic and sauté 1-minute, do not brown garlic. Add the mushrooms and sauté just till the mushroom begin to give off their liquid. Add the brown stock and red wine and bring to a simmer and allow to reduce by 1/3 or until slightly thickened. Remove from the heat and add cold butter, swirl the pan to blend. Serve hot.

Nutrition per Serving
Carbs: 1 g Fiber: 0 g **Net Carbs: 1 g** Protein: trace g Fat: 9 g Calories: 97

Gregory Pryor C.E.C.

Sauces

BBQ Sauce
Servings: 16

1 cup tomato sauce
3 tablespoons Worcestershire sauce
1 tablespoon cider vinegar
1 teaspoon liquid smoke flavoring, or to taste
1 tablespoon Splenda®
1 tablespoon butter

Combine all ingredients and cook over low heat till thick and till flavors blend.

Nutrition per Serving
Carbs: 2 g Fiber: 0 g **Net Carbs: 2 g** Protein: trace g Fat: 1 g Calories: 13

A s we continue with many of the recipes in the entrée section, we will make many more sauce ala' minuet using many of the sauces we have listed so far. From the brown sauce for example we will make mushroom sauce, cracked pepper sauce, brandy sauce and many other pan sauces that we finish with stock and sauces from the above list.

SOUPS

I cannot even begin to emphasize the satisfaction I get from both preparing a great soup and eating a great soup. No matter what the time of year or the occasion, when the mood strikes for soup, few if any other substitute will satisfy this craving. Well Low Carb does not preclude us from enjoying a wide array of bountifully rich and rewarding soups. I am certain the following recipes will satisfy most every desire one may have when the urge arises. Once again, let me emphasize how important having a great stock and top quality products are to making soup. The old theory of using the old or close to expired food products to make soup is out the door nowadays. A full rich flavored soup is every bit a part of a satisfying culinary experience as is a freshly roasted rack of Lamb. The following are prime examples of these full flavored soups. As you will see the opportunities to mold these soups to your own preferences are endless.

Gregory Pryor C.E.C.

Soups

Asparagus Soup with Basil Cream
Servings: 4-6

3 pounds asparagus; tips cut off and reserved separately, stalks peeled cut crosswise into 1-inch pieces For a thicker and fuller body soup allow the pureed mixture to simmer and reduce to a desired thickness.

3 pounds asparagus see note
2 1/2 cups water
1 small onion, chopped
1 1/2 tablespoons unsalted butter
2 cups chicken stock
BASIL CREAM
1/2 cup heavy cream
1 1/2 cups basil leaves, packed
1/2 teaspoon salt

In a small saucepan simmer asparagus cut stalks in water, covered, 15 minutes. Remove and reserve asparagus pieces with slotted spoon and bring water to a boil Add reserved asparagus tips and cook, uncovered, over high heat until crisp-tender, about 3 minutes. Transfer asparagus tips with slotted spoon to a colander, reserving cooking liquid, and rinse under cold water to stop cooking. Drain tips well. In a 4-quart heavy saucepan cook onions in butter with salt and pepper to taste over moderate heat, stirring until pale golden. Add asparagus stalk pieces, broth, and reserved cooking liquid and simmer, covered, 15 minutes, or until asparagus pieces are tender Make basil cream while soup simmers: In a small saucepan bring cream to a boil and stir in basil and salt. Cook mixture over high heat, stirring, until basil is wilted, about 5 to 10 seconds, and in a blender purée mixture. Return basil cream to small saucepan, simmer and reduce by 1/3.
Purée the soup in a clean blender or food processor in small batches and return to 4-quart saucepan. Season the soup with salt and pepper and heat over moderately low heat, stirring occasionally, until heated through Divide soup among 6 bowls and add asparagus tips, arranging them decoratively. Drizzle basil cream over each serving.

Nutrition per Serving Carbs: 6 g Fiber: 2 g **Net Carbs: 4 g** Protein: 3 g Fat: 8 g Calories: 103

Soups

Bacon Cheese Soup

Servings: 4

4 bacon slices
1/2 onion, chopped
1/2 teaspoon dry mustard
1/4 teaspoon black pepper
2 cups chicken stock
4 teaspoons ThickenThin®
2 cups heavy cream
12 ounces cheddar cheese
1/2 teaspoon paprika

In a large heavy bottom saucepan over medium heat, cook bacon until crisp. Remove and drain on paper towels. Crumble bacon.
Add onion to bacon fat in saucepan; cook 3 minutes, until onion just begins to brown.
Add mustard, pepper and stock or broth. Bring to a boil. Reduce heat to low. Whisk in thickener. Add heavy cream, cheese and paprika; stir until cheese is melted.
Ladle soup into four heated soup bowls. Garnish with crumbled bacon.

Nutrition per Serving
Carbs: 3 g Fiber: 0 g **Net Carbs: 3 g** Protein: 13 g Fat: 38 g Calories: 404

Soups

Boiled Beef Soup
Servings: 4

The carb count for this rich flavored soup broth is nearly zero. So feel free to add to the soup broth some aldente' diced vegetables or sliced mushrooms.

2 pounds pot roast with a marrow bone
Cold water
2 stalks celery chopped
2 parsley roots chopped
2 carrots chopped
1 large yellow onion chopped
3 peppercorns
1 teaspoon salt

Place 2 pounds pot roast with a marrow bone (ask butcher for this) in a large soup kettle. Place enough cold water to cover only. (Too much water makes a weak soup.) Bring it to a boil and skim off impurities. Add 2 stalks celery, 2 parsley roots and 2 carrots. Add a large yellow skinned unpeeled onion, 3 or 4 peppercorns and 1 teaspoon salt. Lower heat and simmer very slowly (to keep your soup clear) for 2-1/2 hrs. Or until meat is tender. Strain the liquid and serve hot. Meat or vegetables are delicious served separately with horseradish or any number of the Low Carb salsas.

Nutrition per Serving
Carbs: 3 g Fiber: 1 g **Net Carbs: 2 g** Protein: 1 g Fat: trace g Calories: 19

Soups

Broccoli Rabe and Garlic Soup
Servings: 4

1 medium bunch broccoli rabe stems cut off, yellow and wilted leaves discarded tops and leaves sliced across into 1/2-inch pieces Variations; for several variations, you can substitute any of the following in the same amount, Swiss chard, arugula, bok choy, or any other firm leafy green.

GARLIC BROTH see recipe
2 1/2 teaspoons coarse salt
1/2 teaspoon black pepper
1 medium Broccoli rabe, see note
1/4 cup lemon juice
1/4 cup parmesan cheese, garnish
Salt and pepper, to taste

In a medium saucepan, combine the garlic broth, salt, and pepper. Stir in the broccoli rabe and return to a boil. Lower the heat and simmer until the broccoli rabe is tender, about 4 minutes.
Remove from the heat and stir in the lemon juice to taste.
Check the seasoning and add salt and pepper, if necessary. Pass grated cheese at the table.

Nutrition per Serving
Carbs: 2 g Fiber: 0 g **Net Carbs: 2 g** Protein: 2 g Fat: 2 g Calories: 27

Soups

Chicken Shitake Mushroom and Onion Soup
Servings: 4

Fish sauce is available at Asian markets and in the Asian foods section of many supermarkets.
As an option to sliced mushroom caps, you may quarter them for a distinctive look.

8 cups chicken stock
10 ounces chicken breast, cooked and diced
6 ounces mushroom caps, stemmed and caps sliced
1 tablespoon gingerroot, minced
3 tablespoons fish sauce, see note
1 tablespoon sesame oil
1/4 teaspoon chili oil
2 cups bok choy, thinly sliced
4 teaspoons rice wine vinegar
2 green onion, sliced

Bring stock, mushrooms and ginger to boil in large pot. Reduce heat and simmer 3 minutes. Add fish sauce, soy sauce, sesame oil and chili oil and simmer 2 minutes.
Add bok choy and simmer until bok choy is tender, about 2 minutes. Stir in rice wine vinegar and chicken. Season soup to taste with salt and pepper.
Ladle soup into bowls. Sprinkle with green onions and serve.

Nutrition per Serving
Carbs: 6 g Fiber: 2 g **Net Carbs: 4 g** Protein: 15 g Fat: 11 g Calories: 217

Soups

Creamy Rich Mushroom Soup
Servings: 4

To make this soup even lower in Carbs, omit the dried mushrooms for net Carb 5 grams per serving.

1 ounce dried porcini mushroom, see note
3 tablespoons unsalted butter
3/4 pound mushrooms sliced or quartered
3 garlic clove, minced
2 tablespoons ThickenThin®
3 cups beef stock
1/2 teaspoon dried thyme
1/4 teaspoon ground nutmeg
1/2 cup heavy cream
Salt and pepper, to taste

In a bowl, cover porcinis with enough hot water to cover; let stand 20 minutes. Strain the soaking liquid; set aside. Rinse the soaked mushrooms; finely chop, and set aside.

Melt butter in a saucepot over medium-high heat. Add onion, button mushroom stems and garlic; cook until onion is golden, about 10 minutes.

Add ThickenThin® mix; stir 2 minutes. Gradually stir in broth, water, reserved porcini liquid, thyme and nutmeg. Bring to a boil; reduce heat, cover and simmer 25 minutes.

Add chopped porcini and sliced button mushroom caps to soup; simmer 5 minutes until softened. Blend half the soup in batches in a blender or food processor; return to pot.

Add cream; simmer 2 minutes to heat through. Season with salt and pepper to taste.

Nutrition per Serving
Carbs: 9 g Fiber: 2 g **Net Carbs: 7 g** Protein: 4 g Fat: 20 g Calories: 241

Gregory Pryor C.E.C.

Soups

Egg Drop Soup
Servings: 4

To add another dimension to this soup, add the juice of one whole lemon, or more to taste, and one 10 ounce package of thawed frozen chopped spinach squeezed of all liquid. This makes a wonderful Lemon Spinach Egg Drop Soup.

4 cups chicken stock
2 tablespoons gingerroot, chopped
2 whole eggs, beaten
Salt and white pepper

Bring stock and ginger to a boil in a small saucepan. Hold a serving spoon face down over the pan and slowly pour the egg over the spoon so it drips in ribbons into the simmering soup.
Add green onions. Remove ginger; serve immediately. For an added dimension to flavor, add a 1 inch piece of lemongrass to the stock and the ginger. Season with salt and pepper to taste.

Nutrition per Serving
Carbs: 2 g Fiber: 0 g **Net Carbs: 2 g** Protein: 4 g Fat: 2 g Calories: 57

Soups

Avgolemeno
Servings: 4

6 cups chicken stock
2 tablespoons water
3 whole eggs
1/2 cup lemon juice
Salt and Pepper to Taste

Heat the stock to a simmer in a large stockpot. In a bowl, beat eggs with 2 Tbsp water and the lemon juice. Spoon broth into egg mixture stirring constantly to prevent curdling. After adding about 5 Tbsp. broth to eggs, add eggs to the broth on the stove simmer stirring constantly. Remove from heat. It should be slightly thick. Taste the soup, if you like a stronger lemon flavor add more lemon to taste.

Nutrition per Serving
Carbs: 4 g Fiber: 0 g **Net Carbs: 4 g** Protein: 6 g Fat: 4 g Calories: 90

Gregory Pryor C.E.C.

Soups

Fisherman's Soup
Servings: 4

You can use a variety of fish for this festive soup. If you prefer not to use lobster, squid is a good substitute-just add at the last minute and cook briefly. Lobster tails, cut on underside with scissors. Use any firm white fish, such as cod, halibut or sea bass, cut into 2" pieces.

3 tablespoons olive oil
1/2 cup celery, finely chopped
2 cloves garlic, finely chopped
1/2 pound plum tomato, peeled and chopped
1/4 cup parsley, chopped
1 tablespoon rosemary, chopped
1/2 teaspoon red pepper flakes
3/4 cup dry white wine
6 cups water
4 lobster tails see note
1 pound cod see note
1/2 pound shrimp, 21-25 deveined
Sea salt, to taste
Chopped fresh parsley, garnish
Extra virgin olive oil, garnish

Heat olive oil in large soup pot over medium-low heat. Add celery and cook 5 minutes. Add garlic and cook 1-minute more.
Stir in tomatoes, parsley, rosemary and red pepper flakes. Cook 2 minutes. Add wine; cook until liquid evaporates.
Add water and bring to a boil. Reduce heat; simmer 20 minutes.
Add lobster tails, cook 4 minutes; add fish and cook 3 more minutes until fish is opaque in center. Add shrimp and cook 3 more minutes.

Nutrition per Serving
Carbs: 6 g Fiber: 1 g **Net Carbs: 5 g** Protein: 85 g Fat: 15 g Calories: 548

Soups/Stocks

Garlic Broth
Servings: 20

This is a base for other soups that can also be served on its own – but consider adding some jalapeno pepper, cilantro, and lime juice; or diced tomato, chopped parsley, matchsticks of zucchini, and thinly sliced basil; cooked green beans and small leaves of spinach; lemongrass, basil leaves, and lime juice; or any other seasoning group that seems enjoyable. This broth freezes well for future use in other soups.

3 garlic bulbs, peeled and smashed
1 tablespoon extra virgin olive oil
Sea salt, to taste
Black pepper, to taste
10 cups chicken stock

Cut the garlic cloves in half lengthwise and, if necessary, remove the green germ growing through the center, smash well.
In a medium saucepan, heat the oil over low heat. Stir in the garlic cloves and cook, stirring often, until the outside of the garlic is translucent and cloves are soft, about 20 minutes. Don't let the garlic brown.
Pour in chicken stock. Bring to a boil. Lower the heat and simmer, uncovered, for 40 minutes. The garlic will be very tender. To enjoy this broth on its own, season with salt and pepper to taste; or use as a stock.

Nutrition per Serving
Carbs: 2 g Fiber: 0 g **Net Carbs: 2 g** Protein: 1 g Fat: 1 g Calories: 26

Gregory Pryor C.E.C.

Soups

Vegetable and Shrimp Hot and Sour Soup
Servings: 4

4 cups chicken stock
1/4 cup rice wine vinegar
2 tablespoons Splenda®
1/4 teaspoon ground red pepper
1/4 teaspoon gingerroot, minced
1 pound raw shrimp, peeled and deveined
1 6-ounce package radishes (1-1/2 cups), sliced
1 1/2 cups shredded spinach leaves
2/3 cup sliced green onions (scallions)

In a large saucepan over medium heat, bring stock to a boil. Stir in vinegar, Splenda®, red pepper and ginger. Add shrimp; cook until shrimp turn pink and curl, 3 to 4 minutes.
Turn off heat; stir in radishes, spinach and green onions. Cover and let stand 2 to 3 minutes before serving.
Garnish with enoki mushrooms, if desired.

Nutrition per Serving
Carbs: 4 g Fiber: 1 g **Net Carbs: 3 g** Protein: 16 g Fat: 2 g Calories: 106

Soups

Laotian Tomato and Shrimp Soup
Servings: 4

1 pound fresh tomatoes
1 tablespoon olive oil
1/2 cup chopped onion
1 teaspoon minced garlic
2 tablespoons soy sauce
1 tablespoon sesame oil
1 teaspoon Splenda®
1 teaspoon gingerroot, minced
1 pound shrimp, peeled and deveined

Use tomatoes held at room temperature until fully ripe. Core and coarsely chop tomatoes (makes about 3 cups). In a large saucepan, heat oil over medium heat until hot. Add onion and garlic; cook and stir until softened, about 5 minutes. Add tomatoes, soy sauce, sesame oil, Splenda® and ginger; bring to a boil. Reduce heat to low; simmer, covered, for 30 minutes. Stir in shrimp and return to a boil. Reduce heat and simmer, covered, until shrimp are cooked through and turn pink, 3 to 5 minutes. Serve garnished with chopped cilantro, if desired.

Nutrition per Serving
Carbs: 9 g Fiber: 2 g **Net Carbs: 7 g** Protein: 25 g Fat: 9 g Calories: 216

Gregory Pryor C.E.C.

Soups

New England Clam Chowder
Servings: 4

1 1/2 cups heavy cream
1/4 pound bacon, chopped
3/8 cup celery, chopped
4 cups chicken stock
8 ounces clam juice, 1 bottle
2 cans chopped clams, juice reserved
3 cups cauliflower floweret, cooked
1 dash Tabasco sauce
1 dash Worcestershire sauce
2 tablespoons unsalted butter cut in 1" cubes

In a small saucepan, cook cream 8-10 minutes over medium heat until volume is reduced by half. In a large heavy saucepan over medium heat, cook bacon until cooked, but not crispy. Add celery to saucepan cook 5 minutes, until softened. Stir in chicken stock, bottled clam juice and reserved clam juice; bring to a simmer. In a blender, puree cooked cauliflower, cream and 1 cup of soup until smooth. Return to saucepan. Stir in clams. Bring soup to a simmer; cook 5 minutes.
Season with Tabasco and Worcestershire sauces. Swirl in butter until incorporated. Serve hot.

Nutrition per Serving
Carbs: 9 g Fiber: 1 g **Net Carbs: 8 g** Protein: 17 g Fat: 27 g Calories: 354

Soups

Shrimp Bisque

Servings: 4

Since most of the shrimp in this recipe are pureed, you can buy the smaller less expensive shrimp.

2 tablespoons unsalted butter
1/4 cup onion, chopped
2 cups clam juice
2 tablespoons ThickenThin®
1 pound cooked shrimp, see note
1/2 teaspoon tarragon, chopped
2 tablespoons tomato paste
3/4 cup heavy cream
3/4 cup water

Melt butter in a heavy medium size saucepan over medium heat. Cook onion 5 minutes, until softened. Stir in clam juice and bring to a boil. Reduce heat and simmer 10 minutes. Stir in thickener; whisk until smooth. Separate 8 shrimp; mix the rest in the pot and cook 1-minute, until heated through. Puree soup in a blender in batches; return to pot. Whisk in tarragon, tomato paste cream and water. Bring to a simmer; cook 3 to 4 minutes for flavors to blend.
Season to taste with salt and pepper. Transfer to bowls; garnish with remaining shrimp.

Nutrition per Serving
Carbs: 8 g Fiber: 1 g **Net Carbs: 7 g** Protein: 12 g Fat: 12 g Calories: 192

Gregory Pryor C.E.C.

Soups

Watercress and Squash Soup
Servings: 4

You can substitute spinach for the watercress, substitute zucchini for squash. For a bit of a peppery flavor, substitute the watercress with arugula. Another version of this soup is to use brown stock in place of chicken for a hearty rich soup.

1 tablespoon butter
1 bunch leeks, white part only, chopped
2 medium summer squash, peeled and diced
4 cups chicken stock
1 bunch watercress, tough stems removed
1/2 cup heavy cream
Salt and pepper, to taste

In a large heavy saucepan, melt the butter over moderately low heat. Add the leeks and cook until softened but not browned, 5 to 7 minutes.
Add the squash, increase the heat to moderately high and sauté for 2 minutes without browning. Add the stock and bring to a boil. Reduce the heat to moderate and simmer until the squash is just tender, about 5 minutes. Add the watercress and simmer for 1-minute longer.
Using a food processor or blender, puree the soup, in batches, until smooth. Add the cream, season with salt and pepper to taste. Heat and serve.

Nutrition per Serving
Carbs: 7 g Fiber: 2 g **Net Carbs: 5 g** Protein: 3 g Fat: 14 g Calories: 184

SALADS

Now here is a subject that could be an entire book in and of itself. For purposes of discussion we will look at three basic types of salads. These being, green salads or tossed, bound salads, which are basically cooked meats, poultry or seafood bound with a dressing (usually mayonnaise or vinaigrette) and vegetable salads. With the combination of all the various types of greens, cooked item's and garnishes, the number of salads we can make is nearly endless. I want to spend some time with you talking about the procedures for not only making these salads, but also the proper techniques we must follow to ensure the salad greens are handled and prepared in the correct manner. This will preserve the appearance, flavor and texture of a green or tossed salad. We will also want to look at the proper cooking of the meat, poultry or fish items to again create the freshest and most flavorful salads possible. The numbers and types of greens available in most regions and seasons are seemingly endless. Here is where using your shopping skills are critical to deciding the right greens for your salad. When shopping for salad greens, always look for greens that are fresh, firm to a gentle squeeze, free of blemishes or yellow spots with little or no damage to the outer leaves. Many greens are now packaged and sold in various blends in an airtight plastic package. These are usually a good choice simply because this offers you the variety of greens with out having to buy each individually. Be cautious of these blends, as many are loaded with shredded carrots which add a lot of Carbs to the salad.

No matter what form you buy the greens for your salad; they all need to be prepared with a few common steps. If buying whole greens store these in the coolest part of your refrigerator, that being the lowest part or the crisper. Greens should be stored between 34 and 40 degrees to ensure freshness. When handling fresh greens especially firm lettuce, I prefer that these be torn and not chopped. An exception to this would be romaine lettuce when we are making a Caesar salad. Once the greens are either torn or cut, we need to do a wash and refresh method to these. Greens that are crisp and firm are mandatory to achieve an enjoyable salad. To wash and refresh simply either fill a large bowl with ice and water, or fill a sink with the same. Plunge the greens into this ice-cold water and gently agitate them a bit to loosen and remove any dirt, sand or other particles. Once this is done, allow them to sit in the cold water for 5 to 10 minutes, during which time they will refresh or return to a firm or crisp texture as they are intended. The greens will float on the top of the water and the dirt or sand will sink to the bottom. Take care not to disturb the water when removing the greens, reintroducing the sand or dirt into the greens.

Now equally important is drying the greens. By the way, this same procedure applies to the packaged greens as well. To dry the greens the best and surest way is to use a salad spinner. Many affordable versions of these can be found in nearly every kitchen store. If a salad spinner is not available to you, as you remove the greens, shake off as much water as possible. Lay the greens on several kitchen towels to drain. Gently blot these with either a clean dry kitchen towel or use paper towels making certain the paper towel do not become so wet that it leaves reminisces of itself on your greens. Now your greens are ready to be used in the salad of your choice. Should you have an abundance of greens beyond what you readily need now, these will store nicely if properly stored for 3 to 5 days. To store the fresh cleaned greens place them in a large zip lock bag with a slightly damp paper towel. Now push down on the bag and remove as much air as possible and seal. Here is a great example of the use of the vacuum sealing kitchen appliance we spoke of earlier. Remember to store these in the lowest spot in the fridge as possible.

Now let's take a little time and review the guidelines and components for making a bound salad.

Preparing a salad from cooked foods is a great way to create flavorful and satisfying salads. These salads can serve as a first course or a meal, with lunch time being a prefect a time for of this type of salad to be used as a complete meal. Typically nearly any cooked meat or seafood may be used in a bound salad, as well as fresh vegetables. When considering the ingredients for a bound salads consider these guidelines:

Choose ingredients whose flavors compliment each other without strong contrast.

Choose ingredients for color. A few colorful ingredients can make a simple appearing salad a work of art. For example add just a few diced red peppers to chicken salad to add a vibrancy of color as well as just a slight touch of sweetness.

For proper appearance. Cut all the ingredients in the same shape and size. If the main ingredient is diced, then dice all the other ingredients. If cut on a bias, again continue this cut with all the other ingredients. No matter the style of cut, it should be small enough to eat with a fork. If the salad is to be used as a filling for canapés be certain the dice or cut is small enough to fit onto a canapé.

Be certain any meat or fish item is fully cooked and chilled before incorporating into the bound salad. Please pay close attention to how you cook the meat or seafood item to assure a moist, tender and flavorful item.

Finally, use dressing sparingly. The dressing is intended to enhance the flavor, bind the salad, but not mask it. Now here is a great example of where flavored mayonnaise works well to enhance flavor. Just imagine the variations to the typical chicken salad you can create.

As mentioned earlier, nearly any meat, poultry or seafood will make a great bound salad. Asian beef salad is an example of using beef. Countless version of chicken or turkey salad can be prepared from simple to complex. When cooking chicken or any simmered or poached item for a salad, take this into consideration. When I cook any product in a liquid, I always prepare a flavored liquid. For example if I am cooking chicken or turkey my cooking liquid consists of chicken stock or broth, some celery stalks and a few pieces of onion, skin and all. This not only adds flavor to the poultry, it also leaves a wonderful stock when strained and cooled for other use. When I cook poultry I bring the item to a simmer only. Never boil poultry. Allow the item to cook to a near complete stage. Turn off the heat and let the poultry sit till cool to the touch. This further flavors the poultry as well as allows the moisture to regain its highest level in the poultry. Remove the poultry and let cool. Strain and store the stock as mentioned before. Any whole or parts of a chicken or turkey can be used for a bound salad. Much the same cooking applies to seafood as well; never boil, always simmer let stand, remove and if the stock is flavorful save it for future use in a soup or sauce. Use these flavorful ingredients to create many salads based on your preferences. I always have some form of bound salad at home, either chicken, tuna, egg or ham salad. These are the most common lunch items I enjoy when I am home. Let's now look at some examples of some satisfying green, bound and vegetable salads.

Salad

Arugula, Prosciutto di Parma Salad
Servings: 4

1 large bunch arugula (about 4 cups)
OR
1 large bunch spinach leaves, stems trimmed (about 4 cups)
4 thin slices Prosciutto di Parma (about 2 ounces), cut in 1/2-inch wide strips
1/2 cup shaved or coarsely grated Parmigiano-Reggiano cheese
2 tablespoons toasted pine nuts
1/4 cup prepared balsamic salad dressing

In a large bowl, combine Arugula, Prosciutto di Parma, cheese and pine nuts. Toss gently with salad dressing to coat completely. Serve immediately.

Nutrition per Serving
Carbs: 1 g Fiber: 0 g **Net Carbs: 1 g** Protein: 34 g Fat: 16 g Calories: 291

Salad

Asian Beef Salad
Servings: 4

1 pound boneless beef sirloin, cut 3/4 inch thick
OR
1 pound top round steak, cut 3/4 inch thick
1/4 cup dry sherry
1/4 cup reduced-sodium soy sauce
3 tablespoons vegetable oil, divided
8 ounces mushrooms, sliced
1 6-ounce package frozen pea pods, defrosted
4 cups lettuce, thinly sliced
Red bell pepper slices (optional)

Cut beefsteak into 1/8-inch thick strips. Combine sherry, and soy sauce: pour over strips, stirring to coat. Heat 2 tablespoons oil in large nonstick skillet over medium high heat.
Add mushrooms and pea pods; cook briefly and reserve.
Drain marinade from beef and reserve. Add remaining oil to skillet.
Stir-fry beef strips (1/2 at a time), 1 to 2 minutes. Return vegetables, beef and marinade to skillet; cook and stir until sauce thickens.
Serve beef mixture over lettuce. Garnish if desired.

Nutrition per Serving
Carbs: 9 g Fiber: 3 g **Net Carbs: 6 g** Protein: 28 g Fat: 21 g Calories: 354

Salad

Asian Coleslaw

Servings: 12

I prefer to use a sweet Asian mirin in place of the soy sauce.
To add a color contrast use red cabbage.

4 cups bok choy, thinly sliced
1 cup cabbage leaves, thinly sliced
1 cup snow pea pod, fresh, thinly sliced
2 tablespoons vegetable oil
1 tablespoon sesame oil
2 tablespoons rice wine vinegar
2 teaspoons soy sauce
2 teaspoons gingerroot, grated
1 teaspoon Splenda®, or to taste
Salt, to taste

Place cabbages in a large bowl; Mix in snow peas.
In a small bowl, mix oils, vinegar, soy sauce, ginger and Splenda®. Pour dressing over salad;
Toss to coat. Season to taste with salt.

Nutrition per Serving
Carbs: 2 g Fiber: 1 g **Net Carbs: 1 g** Protein: 1 g Fat: 3 g Calories: 40

Gregory Pryor C.E.C.

Salad

Avocado and Tomato Salad
Servings: 8

3 cups avocado, diced medium
1 1/2 cups grape or cherry tomatoes
1 1/2 cups cucumber, peeled and diced medium
1/4 cup red onion, diced small
3 1/4 tablespoons fresh cilantro, chopped
1 1/2 teaspoons fresh garlic, minced
2 tablespoons lime juice
1/4 cup olive oil
Salt and fresh black pepper to taste

Gently toss ingredients together and serve on a bed of fresh Bibb lettuce.

Nutrition per Serving
Carbs: 7 g Fiber: 2 g **Net Carbs: 5 g** Protein: 2 g Fat: 14 g Calories: 148

Salad

Basic Coleslaw
Servings: 8

1 cabbage head, halved cored and thinly sliced
1 cup cabbage leaves, purple, and thinly sliced
1 cup mayonnaise
1/2 cup sour cream
2 tablespoons cider vinegar
2 teaspoons Splenda®
1 teaspoon celery seed
1 teaspoon salt, or as needed

Cut cabbage halves in half and thinly slice. Transfer to a large bowl.
In a small bowl, whisk together mayonnaise, sour cream, cider vinegar, Splenda®, celery, and salt.
Pour dressing over cabbages. Mix until thoroughly combined. Refrigerate at least 1 hour before serving for flavors to blend.

Nutrition per Serving
Carbs: 8 g Fiber: 3 g **Net Carbs: 5 g** Protein: 3 g Fat: 27 g Calories: 261

Salad

Basic Egg Salad
Servings: 2-4

For a little more distinct flavor, add 1 rounded teaspoon small capers. Some like sweet pickle relish in the mixture. Try adding a little curry powder. Remember to use your imagination.

8 whole eggs, hard-boiled
1/2 cup mayonnaise
1 tablespoon Dijon mustard
1/2 teaspoon salt
1/4 teaspoon white pepper
1/4 cup celery, finely chopped
1/4 cup green onion, finely chopped

Chop eggs roughly, or push them through the large-holed side of a four-sided box grater.
In a large mixing bowl, mix eggs with mayonnaise, mustard, salt and pepper with a spoon. Stir in chopped green onions and chopped celery.

Nutrition per Serving
Carbs: 4 g Fiber: 1 g **Net Carbs: 3 g** Protein: 26 g Fat: 68 g Calories: 717

Salad

Basic Chicken Salad
Servings: 8

Although this is a basic ratio of chicken to mayonnaise and sour cream as well as a basic amount of diced celery, the ratio you use would be a matter of choice. If you like more celery, add more. A drier or wetter consistency use more or less mayo and sour cream. When I make a chicken, seafood or turkey salad I use a 2 to 1 ratio of mayo to sour cream. You can use boneless skinless breast, bone in and skin on, whole chicken or even quarters if you like a dark meat chicken salad. Try using a flavored mayonnaise; add some chopped nuts in small quantity. Want a little more color? Add a fine dice of sweet red bell peppers. This is one of the most versatile bound salads there is. Look for specials in the chicken case and buy what is on sale or the best priced.

4 pounds boneless chicken, see note
2 cups chicken stock
4 stalks celery, rough cut
1 onion, quartered with skin
1 bay leaf
4 stalks celery, diced
3/4 cup mayonnaise
1/4 cup sour cream
2 tablespoons celery seed
Salt and pepper, to taste

Place chicken, rough cut celery tops and all, onion and bay leaf in a stockpot. Cover with chicken stock.
Bring to a simmer and cook till chicken is cooked nearly through. 12-15 minutes.
Test chicken by cutting a piece to check to be certain no pink color remains.
Turn of heat and let chicken sit in stockpot till cool to the touch.
While chicken is cooling, slice the remaining celery in thirds and dice.
Once chicken is cool enough to handle, remove and drain chicken. Cut chicken into approx. 1/4 x 1/4 or 3/8 x 3/8 dice. Add diced celery. Add mayonnaise and sour cream. Stir to coat and mix well. Add celery seed and season to taste with salt and pepper.

Nutrition per Serving
Carbs: 2 g Fiber: 1 g **Net Carbs: 1 g** Protein: 54 g Fat: 23 g Calories: 437

Salad

Cobb Salad

Servings: 4

This is the basic recipe, you may improvise with any Low Carb veggies you have.
If you like, omit the dressing in this recipe, and use one of many included in this book.

3 cups romaine lettuce, chopped
3 cups iceberg lettuce, chopped
1 pound chicken breast, cooked and diced
1/2 pound bacon, cooked and crumbled
1 tomato, seeded and chopped
4 green onion, chopped
1/4 cup red wine vinegar
1 teaspoon Dijon mustard
1/2 cup olive oil
1 avocado, peeled and sliced
3/4 cup blue cheese, crumbled
1 egg, hard-boiled

In a large bowl, mix Romaine and iceberg lettuces, chicken, bacon, tomato, and green onions.
In a small bowl, whisk vinegar, mustard, until combined. Slowly whisk in olive oil. Pour 3/4 of the dressing over salad and mix well.
Divide salad on 4 plates.
Sprinkle cheese and chopped eggs over salads. Arrange avocado slices on top; drizzle with remaining dressing.

Nutrition per Serving
Carbs: 10 g Fiber: 3 g **Net Carbs: 7 g** Protein: 46 g Fat: 80 g Calories: 936

Salad

Cucumber Tomato Salad
Servings: 4

2 cucumbers
3 tablespoons red wine vinegar
2 teaspoons Splenda®
1/2 teaspoon salt
3 roma tomatoes
1/2 cup green onion, chopped
1/4 cup fresh basil leaves, chopped
2 tablespoons olive oil
Black pepper, to taste

Peel cucumber, cut in half lengthwise and scoop out seeds with a small spoon. Cut cucumber into ½" slices and transfer to a large serving bowl. Toss with vinegar, Splenda® and salt. Let sit 30 minutes Add tomatoes, green onions, basil and olive oil to bowl. Gently mix to combine all ingredients. Season to taste with additional salt and pepper.

Nutrition per Serving
Carbs: 10 g Fiber: 3 g **Net Carbs: 7 g** Protein: 2 g Fat: 7 g Calories: 104

Salad

Ham Salad
Servings: 4

Any cooked ham is fine for this recipe. If you don't have a grinder, ask the deli to grind the ham for you. Alternately you can cut the ham into large chunks and using a food processor with a pulse action grind the ham. Or chop with a knife to a fine minced texture.

1 pound ham, see notes
2 tablespoons Dijon mustard
3 tablespoons mayonnaise or as needed to combine to desired consistency
1 green onion, finely chopped
1 tablespoon dill pickle, finely chopped

In a mixing bowl, combine ham, mustard, and mayonnaise. Mix well. Stir in green onion and pickle. Chill at least 1-hour.

Nutrition per Serving
Carbs: 4 g Fiber: 0 g **Net Carbs: 4 g** Protein: 20 g Fat: 21 g Calories: 288

Salad

Mock Potato Salad
Servings: 4

2 cups cauliflower flowerets
1/2 cup mayonnaise
2 tablespoons lemon juice
1/2 teaspoon mustard
3 green onions, chopped
2 tablespoons green bell pepper, chopped
1/4 cup celery, chopped
1 teaspoon celery seed
2 eggs, hard-boiled copped
Salt and pepper, to taste

Cook cauliflower in a large pot of boiling salted water 10 minutes, until tender. Drain and rinse under cold water; pat dry. In a large mixing bowl, mix mayonnaise, lemon juice and mustard. Add cauliflower, eggs, green onion and green pepper, if using. Mix well until vegetables are evenly coated with dressing. Add salt and pepper to taste. Chill 1-hour to allow flavors to blend.

Nutrition per Serving
Carbs: 5 g Fiber: 2 g **Net Carbs: 3 g** Protein: 5 g Fat: 26 g Calories: 259

Salad

Salad of Ahi Tuna Seared with Lavender and Pepper with Whole Grain Mustard Sauce

Servings: 4

Tip; to ensure a smooth clean slice, wrap Tuna tightly in plastic wrap. Slice through the plastic wrap making certain all the plastic wrap is removed after slicing.

1 teaspoon black peppercorns
2 teaspoons fennel seeds
1 teaspoon white peppercorns
2 teaspoons sea salt
1 teaspoon dried lavender flowers
1 1/2 pounds tuna steak, Ahi sushi grade
For Mustard Sauce
2 ounces whole grain mustard
1 ounce olive oil
1 teaspoon mustard seed, toasted
1 teaspoon rice wine vinegar
1 teaspoon Splenda®
8 ounces mixed greens

Using a mortar and pestle or a rolling pin, crush the ingredients for the lavender-pepper coating.
Lightly oil the tuna with 2 teaspoons of olive oil; coat lightly and evenly with the lavender-pepper mixture.
Heat the remaining oil in a skillet to just the smoking point and quickly sear the tuna on all sides. This should not take more than 2 minutes. Immediately chill the tuna.
Mix the ingredients for the mustard sauce. Set aside.
To serve, thinly slice the tuna into 3 or 4 1/8 inch medallions per serving. Arrange on a chilled plate with baby greens and a small dollop of the mustard sauce.

Nutrition per Serving
Carbs: 6 g Fiber: 3 g **Net Carbs: 3 g** Protein: 42 g Fat: 16 g Calories: 339

129

Gregory Pryor C.E.C.

Salad

Seven Layer Salad
Servings: 4 entrée or 8 sides

DRESSING
1/2 cup mayonnaise
3/4 cup sour cream
OR
3/4 cup yogurt
1/4 cup parsley, chopped
1/2 teaspoon cayenne pepper
2 teaspoons Worcestershire sauce
1 teaspoon garlic, chopped fine
2 teaspoons Splenda®
SALAD
3 cups cabbage, shredded
2 cups broccoli stalks, grated
1 cup celery, grated
2 cups cauliflower, cut small
1/4 cup bacon (approximately 6 ounces raw), cooked and crumbled

Combine all ingredients for dressing. In glass bowl, layer cabbage and broccoli, then spread 1/3 of dressing over layered vegetables.
Continue to layer celery and cauliflower. Spread remaining dressing over cauliflower and refrigerate at least 2 hours, preferably overnight. Sprinkle with bacon and serve.

Nutrition per Serving
Carbs: 7 g Fiber: 2 g **Net Carbs: 5 g** Protein: 6 g Fat: 21 g Calories: 227

Salad

Shrimp and Cucumber Salad

Servings: 4

1 cucumber, small
1 pound shrimp, 21-25
1/4 cup rice wine vinegar
1 tablespoon Splenda®
1 tablespoon soy sauce
1 tablespoon fresh gingerroot, grated
1 tablespoon sesame seeds, toasted

Peel the cucumber and halve it lengthways and remove any seeds with a teaspoon. Cut the cucumber into thin slices, sprinkle with salt and set aside for 5 minutes. Rinse to remove the salt and pat dry with a paper towel. Place the shrimp in a pan of slightly salted water and simmer for about 2-3 minutes, or until just cooked. Drain the shrimp and plunge them into a bowl of ice water. When cool, peel and devein the shrimp leaving the tails intact.

Place the vinegar, Splenda®, soy sauce and ginger in a glass bowl and stir till the Splenda® is dissolved.

Add the cucumbers and shrimp and marinate in the refrigerator for at least 1-hour.

Toast the seeds in a dry pan, drain the cucumbers and shrimp and serve cold with the toasted seeds sprinkled over-the-top of the shrimp and cucumbers.

Nutrition per Serving
Carbs: 5 g Fiber: 1 g **Net Carbs: 4 g** Protein: 24 g Fat: 3 g Calories: 149

Gregory Pryor C.E.C.

Salad

Thai Style Cold Lobster Salad
Servings: 4

2 pounds spiny lobster, whole, cooked
2 tablespoons minced fresh cilantro
Lettuce leaves
DRESSING
1 tablespoon light oil
1 clove garlic, pressed or minced
2 tablespoons rice vinegar
1/2 tablespoon light soy sauce
1/2 tablespoon toasted sesame seeds
1 tablespoon green onions or chives, minced
1/4 teaspoon fresh ginger, minced
1/8 teaspoon pepper
Juice of 1 lime

Remove lobster meat from shell and cut into chunks. Blend dressing ingredients together, then toss with lobster meat and chill. Serve on lettuce leaves; garnish with cilantro.

Nutrition per Serving
Carbs: 2 g Fiber: 0 g **Net Carbs: 2 g** Protein: 43 g Fat: 6 g Calories: 244

Salad

Wilted Spinach Salad with Roasted Peppers

Servings: 6

1 red pepper
2 ounces extra virgin olive oil
1/2 red onion, thinly sliced
4 cups fresh spinach
1 escarole head, small
1 clove garlic, finely chopped
12 pitted ripe olives
1 ounce parmesan cheese, grated
Salt and pepper, to taste

Roast, peel and cut the peppers into ¼ inch strips. Toss the peppers with ½ tablespoon of olive oil and a few pinches of salt and pepper. Set aside to marinate.

Cover the onion slices with cold water to leach the strong onion flavor. Set aside.

Stem, wash and dry the spinach. Trim the stem end of the escarole and discard the tough outer leaves. Wash and dry.

Drain the onions. In a large bowl, combine the vinegar, garlic, ½ teaspoon salt and a few pinches of pepper. Add the greens, onion, peppers and olives.

Heat the remaining olive oil in a small pan until very hot and just below the smoking point. Immediately pour it over the salad and toss with a pair of metal tongs or two forks to coat and wilt the leaves. Sprinkle on the Parmesan Cheese and divide into equal portions

Nutrition per Serving
Carbs: 7 g Fiber: 3 g **Net Carbs: 4 g** Protein: 4 g Fat: 12 g Calories: 146

T his is only the tip of the iceberg (no pun intended) in the total scheme of salads. I encourage you again to use your imagination to expand the array of salads. Consider the simplicity of Tomato, Basil and Mozzarella Cheese with Extra Virgin Olive oil. Simply mix mayonnaise, cooked chicken, diced celery, add some curry powder and you have Curry Chicken Salad. Shrimp, Crab, Squid, the sky is the limit in your creation of simple to complex salads.

How here are a few salad dressings to use in your Low Carb Lifestyle salads.

Salad Dressing

Balsamic Vinaigrette

Servings: 8

1 1/2 Cup extravirgin olive oil
1/2 Cup balsamic vinegar
3/4 teaspoon minced garlic
3/4 teaspoon Splenda®
1/8 teaspoon salt

In a bowl whisk olive oil, vinegar, garlic, Splenda® and salt until blended.
Yield: 2 Tablespoons per serving

Nutrition per Serving
Carbs: 1 g Fiber: 0 g **Net Carbs: 1 g** Protein: trace g Fat: 14 g Calories: 124

Salad Dressing

Emulsified Vinaigrette Dressing

Servings: 8

The flavor of this dressing can be altered to match any desire. Add ¼ cup pureed basil for a basil version. Increase the lemon for a stronger lemon dressing. Let your imagination guide you.

2 whole eggs
1 tablespoon salt
1/2 teaspoon white pepper
1 tablespoon paprika
1 tablespoon dry mustard
1 tablespoon Splenda®
1 pinch cayenne pepper
4 ounces cider vinegar
24 ounces salad oil or olive oil for a nuttier flavor
4 ounces lemon juice

Place the whole eggs in the bowl of a mixer (kitchen aide) and whip on high-speed until eggs are frothy. Add the dry ingredients and about 1 ounce of vinegar, continue to whip. With mixer on high, slowly begin adding oil in a steady stream. As needed add a little vinegar to thin the emulsion. Continue to add the oil in a steady stream till all the oil, vinegar and lemon juice is added. Season to taste.

Nutrition per Serving
Carbs: 2 g Fiber: 0 g **Net Carbs: 2 g** Protein: trace g Fat: 6 g Calories: 59

Gregory Pryor C.E.C.

Salad Dressing

Blue Cheese Salad Dressing
Servings: 8

Feel free to substitute gorgonzola cheese if you so desire.
Save those empty mayonnaise jars for your fresh salad dressings.
Be certain to taste this dressing and adjust seasoning, be careful not to add any salt till you taste this, as blue cheese tends to be a bit salty.

1 cup mayonnaise
1 cup sour cream
6 ounces crumbled bleu cheese
1/4 cup olive oil
1 tablespoon buttermilk
1 teaspoon red wine vinegar
1 clove garlic, optional
1/4 teaspoon dry mustard
1/2 teaspoon white pepper

Combine all ingredients in a small bowl; stir until well blended. Cover and chill.

Nutrition per Serving
Carbs: 2 g Fiber: 0 g **Net Carbs: 2 g** Protein: 6 g Fat: 42 g Calories: 396

Salad Dressing

Classic Ranch Dressing

Servings: 8

Although classically garlic is used in ranch dressing, you may omit this if you desire a garlic free dressing.

3/4 cup mayonnaise
1/2 cup buttermilk
2 tablespoons parsley, chopped
3/4 teaspoon onion powder
1 clove garlic, chopped
1 teaspoon Dijon mustard
1 teaspoon lemon juice

Combine all ingredients in a blender; puree until smooth. Season to taste with salt and pepper.

Nutrition per Serving
Carbs: 1 g Fiber: 0 g **Net Carbs: 1 g** Protein: 1 g Fat: 18 g Calories: 156

Salad Dressing

Easy Caesar Salad Dressing

Servings: 8

Adjust the garlic to your individual taste.
You can omit the anchovies if you so desire, but the flavor will suffer.

2 cups mayonnaise
2 2-ounce cans anchovies, drained
1/4 cup Dijon-style mustard
1/4 cup fresh lemon juice
4 cloves garlic, or to taste
1/4 cup parmesan cheese, shredded
1 teaspoon ground white pepper

In a blender or food processor, blend ingredients.

Nutrition per Serving
Carbs: 2 g Fiber: 0 g **Net Carbs: 2 g** Protein: 6 g Fat: 49 g Calories: 446

Gregory Pryor C.E.C.

Salad Dressing

Green Goddess Dressing
Servings: 4 - 6

Anchovy paste makes this dressing special; however you can omit this if the idea of anchovy does not sit well with you.

1/2 cup mayonnaise
1/2 cup sour cream
1 tablespoon white wine vinegar
1/4 cup parsley, chopped
2 tablespoons green onions
1 tablespoon fresh tarragon, chopped
1 teaspoon anchovy paste, optional
Salt and pepper, to taste

Process all ingredients, with 2 tablespoons of water in a food processor or blender until smooth. Add salt and pepper to taste.

Nutrition per Serving
Carbs: 2 g Fiber: 0 g **Net Carbs: 2 g** Protein: 2 g Fat: 30 g Calories: 265

Salad Dressing

Thousand Island Dressing
Servings: 16

I recommend using the Mt Olive no sugar pickles, and grinding or chopping your own relish.

1 tablespoon red wine vinegar
1 tablespoon Splenda®
2 cups mayonnaise
1/4 cup Low Carb ketchup
1/4 cup sweet pickle relish, no sugar added
4 eggs, hard-boiled, chopped
2 tablespoons parsley, chopped
1 bunch green onion, chopped
Salt and pepper to taste
Worcestershire sauce to taste

In a large mixing bowl combine the vinegar and Splenda® to dissolve the Splenda®.
Add the remaining ingredients, mix well and season to taste.

Nutrition per Serving
Carbs: trace g Fiber: 0 g **Net Carbs: trace g** Protein: 2 g Fat: 25 g Calories: 222

Gregory Pryor C.E.C.

Condiments

Tomato Ketchup

Save carbs and money with this easy condiment recipe.

7 pounds ripe tomatoes (about 21 medium)
1 cup Splenda®
1/2 cup coarsely chopped hot red pepper optional
1 piece (3 inches) cinnamon stick, broken in pieces
1/2 teaspoon whole cloves
1 cup cider vinegar
1 1/2 teaspoons paprika
1 teaspoon salt

Rinse tomatoes; plunge into boiling water, then into cold water. Peel and quarter, removing as many seeds as possible. Force tomatoes through sieve or food mill. (There should be roughly 2 quarts of pulp.) Combine pulp in large pot with vinegar, Splenda® and salt. Tie remaining ingredients loosely in cheesecloth bag and add to tomato mixture. Bring to boil over medium heat; reduce heat and simmer 1-hour, or until ketchup is of desired consistency.
Stir occasionally to prevent sticking. Remove cheesecloth bag. If ketchup appears a bit chunky puree in a food processor. Ladle into clean, hot jars. Seal, follow manufacturer's directions. Process in boiling water bath 5 minutes.

Nutrition per Serving
Carbs: 3 g Fiber: 1 g **Net Carbs: 2 g** Protein: 1 g Fat: 0 g Calories: 14

I hope these examples have inspired you to become creative in respect to the endless array of salad variations that you can include in your Low Cab lifestyle. I know they play a big part in my day-to-day needs.

Now I want to move to those great side dishes. You know that round off the dinner plate next to the exquisite entrée's we will be getting too soon. When we get into the many side dishes that fit into our Low Carb Lifestyle, one has to only think, *"Keep it simple"*. Now what do I mean by that? Basically this; most every side dish that we choose to offer to go with our entrée should be colorful, flavorful and compliment the entrée. To accomplish this we don't have to spend a lot of time doing so, nor does it make sense that you should have to. When we use fresh quality produce and a few simple techniques these, typically vegetables are transformed into just what they are intended to be, a *"side dish"*. I cannot tell you how many times in a restaurant I have ask for the vegetable of the day, and been so disappointed in knowing that once this fresh vegetable had the opportunity to be such a nice product, but instead it was served to me either nearly raw, or worse cooked to near mush, bland and unseasoned. Doesn't that just ruin the meal? Of course it does. And why?

To make a flavorful side dish is simple. Take for example; Fresh green beans, blanched to just tender, and tossed in a sauté pan of browned butter with salt and pepper. Simple, colorful and flavorful. This same simple technique can be used for nearly any fresh vegetable. Consider either cauliflower or broccoli floweret's again steamed or blanched till just crisp tender and tossed in browned butter with seasoning, how difficult is that? Or those same flowerets well seasoned and served with a cheese sauce. I tell most apprentice cooks that have been under my supervision *"don't try to impress me with being able to grille a steak, impress me with your vegetable cooking skills"*. Nowadays it seems everyone either serves bland over or uncooked vegetables and this just boggles my mind. It's so easy to do them right, and above all not to mention the nutritional values. It just makes the meal so much more complete when all parts of the meal are done correctly. Another simple favorite of mine is a julienne of zucchini and summer squash tossed in hot olive oil. Add a little chopped basil at the end season to taste and that's it. Simple, colorful and flavorful. Again, my whole point in all this is right back to the earlier part of this book. This lifestyle is not boring, it should be simple, and with a little creativity anyone can and will cook like a professional in your own kitchen. Here is a simple tip, if you didn't already know this. To set the color of a vegetable, to the water you intend to blanch the vegetable add 1 teaspoon of white vinegar and always bring the water or stock to a boil before adding the vegetable. For example; when I intend to serve freshly sautéed green beans, I always use either chicken stock or broth to blanch them in. Use the following recipes as a guide to get those creative juices flowing.

VEGETABLES AND SIDE DISHES

Side Dishes

Braised Brussel Sprouts with Dill
Servings: 4

If using fresh follow cooking times. You can substitute frozen. Thaw if using frozen and reduce cooking time in the first step to 4 minutes.

1 pound brussel sprout
2 tablespoons white wine vinegar
1 cup chicken stock
1/4 cup dill weed, fresh, chopped
Salt and pepper, to taste

Trim sprouts; halve if desired. In large pot of boiling salted water, cook brussel sprouts for 8 minutes if whole, 6 minutes if halved, or until barely tender.
Drain, refresh under cold running water and drain. In a well buttered casserole, combine sprouts, vinegar, dill, stock and salt and pepper to taste; mix well.
Bake, covered in 350 degree oven for 10 minutes. Uncover and bake for 5 minutes longer.

Nutrition per Serving
Carbs: 10 g Fiber: 4 g **Net Carbs: 6 g** Protein: 4 g Fat: trace g Calories: 51

Side Dishes

Braised Celery
Servings: 4

I like to use celery as often as possible in many ways. It is low in net carbs and a great source of fiber.
This is a simple dish to prepare and certain to be a favorite to go with any entree'.
Cooking time will vary depending on the size of the celery heads. The celery should be tender when checked with a fork. Serve each half as one serving.

2 celery whole heads
1 bay leaf
1 tablespoon white vinegar
3 cups chicken stock
Salt and pepper, to taste

Remove the leafy tops from each head of celery. Leaving the root end intact, cut each lengthwise in half.
Wash well to remove any grit. Place each half (4) in a baking dish. Add bay leaf and vinegar and stock. Cover and bake in a 350 degree oven for approx 40 minutes. Celery should be tender.
Remove and hold covered to keep warm. Reduce the cooking liquid till thick and spoon lightly over celery at service.

Nutrition per Serving
Carbs: 2 g Fiber: 1 g **Net Carbs: 1 g** Protein: 1 g Fat: trace g Calories: 20

Side Dishes

Broccoli with Lemon and Garlic

Servings: 4

A simple twist to basic steamed broccoli.

2 cups broccoli florets
2 cloves garlic, minced
3 tablespoons extra virgin olive oil
3 tablespoons lemon juice, fresh
Salt and pepper, to taste

Steam broccoli till tender but firm, 6-8 minutes. Meanwhile, mince the garlic. Heat the oil in a nonstick skillet over medium heat; add the garlic sauté one minute.
Add the cooked broccoli, lemon juice and salt and pepper to taste, toss the broccoli to mix. Cooking briefly to heat through.

Nutrition per Serving
Carbs: 3 g Fiber: 1 g **Net Carbs: 2 g** Protein: 1 g Fat: 10 g Calories: 105

Side Dishes

Creamed Spinach 1

Servings: 4

Basic and simple. If you should desire, I like to add to this recipe one fine diced shallot that has been sweated in a small amount of butter.

2 10-ounce package frozen chopped spinach
1 3-ounce package cream cheese, softened
1 tablespoon melted butter
1/8 teaspoon ground nutmeg
1 tablespoon Parmesan cheese

Cook spinach according to package directions; drain well. Stir together cream cheese, butter and nutmeg. Stir in spinach, spoon into lightly greased 1-quart casserole, sprinkle with Parmesan cheese. Cover and bake at 350°F oven for 20 minutes.

Nutrition per Serving
Carbs: 3 g Fiber: 2 g **Net Carbs: 1 g** Protein: 4 g Fat: 11 g Calories: 123

Gregory Pryor C.E.C.

Side Dishes

Creamed Spinach 2
Servings: 4

This simple version can be finished in one saucepan or larger sauté pan. By thawing the spinach before use you can remove most of the water by squeezing the spinach nearly dry.

2 10-ounce package frozen chopped spinach thawed and squeezed dry
1 tablespoon melted butter
1 shallot chopped fine
1 tablespoon butter
3 ounces shredded Swiss cheese
1/4 cup heavy cream
1/8 teaspoon ground nutmeg
1 tablespoon Parmesan cheese

Melt the butter in a saucepan or large sauté pan over medium heat, Add the shallot and sweat just till tender. Add spinach and heat through. Add cream, cheeses and nutmeg and cook till cheese melts and the spinach and sauce thicken.

Nutrition per Serving
Carbs: 4 g Fiber: 2 g **Net Carbs: 2 g** Protein: 4 g Fat: 11 g Calories: 123

Side Dish

Garlic Green Beans

Servings: 4

1 pounds green beans, cleaned and ends removed
1 tablespoon salt
1 tablespoon olive oil
2 teaspoons garlic, minced
1/4 cup basil, chopped fresh
Salt and pepper to taste

Bring a large pot of water or chicken stock to a boil. Add one tablespoon of salt. Drop cleaned beans into pot. Cook green beans until tender, yet firm. Remove from pot and pour cold water over beans until they are cool.
Heat large sauté pan, add oil and beans. Cook 3-4 minutes. Add garlic and basil and continue to cook until beans are hot. Season with salt and pepper.

Nutrition per Serving
Carbs: 9 g Fiber: 5 g **Net Carbs: 4 g** Protein: 2 g Fat: 2 g Calories: 60

Gregory Pryor C.E.C.

Side Dish

Green Beans with Red Pepper Julienne and Basil

Servings: 4

1 pounds green beans, cleaned and ends removed
1 Red Bell Pepper cut into julienne seeds and membrane removed
1 bunch fresh clean basil chopped or chiffonade
1 tablespoon salt
1 tablespoon olive oil
2 teaspoons garlic, minced optional
1/4 cup basil, chopped fresh
Salt and pepper to taste

Bring a large pot of water or chicken stock to a boil. Add one tablespoon of salt. Drop cleaned beans into pot. Cook green beans until tender, yet firm. Remove from pot and pour cold water over beans until they are cool. In same pot add the peppers and blanch for approx 3 minutes. Remove and rinse under cold water.
Heat large sauté pan, add oil, peppers and beans. Cook 3-4 minutes. Add garlic and basil and continue to cook until beans are hot. Season with salt and pepper.

Nutrition per Serving
Carbs: 11 g Fiber: 6 g **Net Carbs: 5 g** Protein: 2 g Fat: 2 g Calories: 60

Side Dish

Grilled Spirited Mushrooms
Servings: 4

1 pound small to medium-sized fresh white mushrooms
2 tablespoons olive oil
1/2 teaspoon salt
1/4 teaspoon ground black pepper
3 tablespoons butter
1 teaspoon finely chopped fresh garlic
1/4 cup dry sherry
1/4 cup chopped fresh parsley

Preheat grill or broiler. Trim mushroom stems; halve mushrooms. In a medium bowl, combine oil, salt and pepper; add mushrooms and toss well. Transfer mushrooms to a vegetable grate or rack in a broiler pan; grill or broil until lightly browned and softened, turning occasionally, about 5 minutes. Meanwhile, in a medium saucepan, melt butter. Add garlic; cook and stir until softened and pale gold, about 1-minute. Add sherry; simmer for 1-minute. Stir in mushrooms and parsley; toss well. Serve over grilled hamburgers, grilled steaks or as a side dish.

Nutrition per Serving
Carbs: 4 g Fiber: 1 g **Net Carbs: 3 g** Protein: 2 g Fat: 11 g Calories: 122

Gregory Pryor C.E.C.

Side Dish

Grilled Marinated Portabella Mushrooms
Servings: 4
Often called the Beef of the vegetable world.

4 large Portobello mushroom caps
1 cup beef stock
2 tablespoons shallots, minced
2 tablespoons fresh garlic, chopped
1/4 cup olive oil
1 tablespoon fresh rosemary, chopped
1/2 teaspoon dried thyme
Salt and pepper, to taste

Place mushrooms in a shallow pan; combine remaining ingredients and pour over-the-top of the mushrooms.
Marinate for 1-2 hours, turning once. Remove from marinade and cook on hot grill for 3 minutes on each side.
Slice and serve as a side dish or main course.

Nutrition per Serving
Carbs: 6 g Fiber: 2 g **Net Carbs: 4 g** Protein: 3 g Fat: 14 g Calories: 166

Side Dish

Grilled Vegetables
Servings: 4

MARINADE
1/2 cup red wine vinegar
1 1/2 cups olive oil
2 cloves fresh garlic, minced
1 tablespoon fresh rosemary, chopped
1 tablespoon fresh oregano, chopped
1 tablespoon fresh basil, chopped
1 tablespoon fresh parsley, chopped
1 tablespoon Splenda®
Salt and fresh ground black pepper to taste
1 small zucchini, sliced 3/4 inch thick
1 small to medium yellow squash, sliced 3/4 inch thick
1 Japanese eggplant, sliced 3/4 inch thick

Combine all ingredients for marinade and pour over sliced vegetables, marinate for 30 minutes. Cook on a hot grill for 2-3 minutes on each side.
As an alternate to grilling, this also is excellent if you wish to sauté this dish in hot olive oil in a large sauté pan.

Nutrition per Serving
Carbs: 6 g Fiber: 2 g **Net Carbs: 4 g** Protein: 1 g Fat: 26 g Calories: 383

Gregory Pryor C.E.C.

Side Dish

Garden Ratatouille
Servings: 4

1 tablespoon olive oil
1/2 medium onion, chopped
1 clove garlic, minced
1 medium green bell pepper, thinly sliced
1 medium red bell pepper, thinly sliced
1 cup sliced fresh mushrooms
1 medium zucchini, thinly sliced
1/2 medium eggplant, peeled and cubed
2 tablespoons minced fresh basil
1 1/2 cups Low Carb Tomato Sauce
1/3 cup grated Parmesan cheese

Preheat oven to 400 degrees F.
In a large skillet, heat 2 tablespoons oil over medium heat. Add onion, garlic, green and red peppers, and mushrooms. Sauté until vegetables are tender. Remove and set aside.
Sauté zucchini and eggplant, adding more oil as needed. Return sautéed pepper mixture to skillet. Add basil and sauce; simmer 5 minutes over low heat, stirring occasionally.
Spoon vegetable mixture into shallow baking dish. Evenly sprinkle with cheese. Bake covered, 25-30 minutes or until bubbly.

Nutrition per Serving
Carbs: 11 g Fiber: 4 g **Net Carbs: 7 g** Protein: 5 g Fat: 6 g Calories: 109

Side Dish

Mock Mashed Potatoes

Servings: 4

These mock mashed potatoes are so close to real, you will never miss the real ones again. Add any flavors to these such as, horseradish, roasted garlic or any other taste you have been missing in mashed potatoes.
You can process these in a food processor, but take care not to over process and make this to liquid.
Here is a real tip. For that thick fluffy mashed potato texture. Before mashing the cauliflower, in a kitchen aide or food processor, whip 1/8 cup of heavy cream to hard stiff peaks, add the cauliflower and whip till smooth. Season and flavor as you normally would.

1 large head cauliflower or 2 small
4 ounces cream cheese
1 tablespoon butter
Salt and pepper, to taste

Clean cauliflower of all outer leaves and the larger stalks. Cut into pieces. Cook cauliflower in boiling salted water till soft.
Remove from pot and drain. Put cauliflower in a large bowl or the bowl of a Kitchen Aide appliance.
Either beat or whip cauliflower till smooth. Add cream cheese and blend well. Finish with butter and season to taste with salt and pepper.

Nutrition per Serving
Carbs: 2 g Fiber: 1 g **Net Carbs: 1 g** Protein: 3 g Fat: 13 g Calories: 131

Gregory Pryor C.E.C.

Side Dish

Sautéed Greens
Servings: 4

Any good quality fresh greens work well for this dish, I enjoy Red Swiss chard above all others. Sautéed greens are one of my favorite side dishes for several reasons. The variations of greens allow variety. They are easily prepared, and can be seasoned or flavored in many ways. For example fry and crumble some bacon, then sauté the greens in the bacon drippings, splash with flavored vinegar at the end for added flavor. And best of all these are another great Low Carb source of fiber.

1 1/2 pounds Fresh greens (Swiss chard, mustard, turnip or spinach), chopped
2 tablespoons olive or vegetable oil
2 tablespoons garlic (optional), chopped
Salt and pepper, to taste

Trim the stems from the greens. Soak in lots of cool water to wash away the sand. Shake the water from the greens and dry them. They must be dry when they are cooked.
Place oil in a wide and heavy sauté pan. Add garlic to the pan. Stir, then immediately add greens (all at once if possible). Stir continuously for about 5 minutes. Season with salt and pepper and serve.

Nutrition per Serving
Carbs: 7 g Fiber: 5 g **Net Carbs: 2 g** Protein: 4 g Fat: 3 g Calories: 62

Side Dishes

Asparagus Quiche
Servings: 12

This is a basic Quiche. Any Low Carb item may be added, such as broccoli, spinach, ham, etc. Use your Low Carb imagination to create a special Quiche for any occasion.

1 cup shredded Swiss cheese
1/2 cup shredded Cheddar cheese
1 cup chopped asparagus
1/4 cup chopped leeks
1/2 cup sliced mushrooms
12 whole eggs
1 cup milk
1 cup whipping cream
Nutmeg, to taste
Pepper, to taste

Preheat oven to 375º degrees. Grease a deep dish pie pan or 10 "× 10" Pyrex pan. Spread cheese on bottom of pan and top with vegetables.
Whisk together eggs, milk, cream, nutmeg and pepper. Pour over cheese and vegetables. Bake about 45 minutes or until knife inserted in center comes out clean.

Nutrition per Serving
Carbs: 3 g Fiber: 0 g **Net Carbs: 3 g** Protein: 11 g Fat: 17 g Calories: 205

LOW CARB WRAPS

How fortunate for us that we now have a great tasting and versatile product available in Low Carb. For many people that I know this addition to the Low Carb products has replaced that occasion to make a sandwich. For many years Wraps have been and in many places are considered a most trendy lunch time meal. As of now these items are in limited retail locations. However, they are readily available by either mail order or via the internet. Look for these soon in a retail market (they are becoming a popular item). The Low Carb Tortilla is the La Tortilla Factory brand and may be purchased either by calling 707 586-4000 or by visiting them on the internet at http://www.latortillafactory.com/index.htm. The following suggestions are not specific in recipe form. The varieties of Wraps one could create is so endless that all you need to do is use that Low Carb thinking. I have offered here a few suggestions, in addition to the many ideas they offer for Wraps on their web site. I offered wraps during the Spring and Summer seasons at the Country Club and these are but a few of the typical Wraps we offered at various times. Think about your own possible creations. Choose any of the Low Carb Salads in this book or any of your own, and simply spread evenly on a Tortilla and wrap it up. I also suggest that you lightly toast the Tortilla. Considering a net Carb of 3 grams per Tortilla, by being responsible with the fillings you can easily have a 6-7 Gram lunch and be fully satisfied. Now take a look at these suggestions and be prepared to fall in love with wraps.

CAESAR WRAP
Romaine Lettuce
Parmesan Cheese
Mozzarella cheese
Chopped tomatoes
Sliced olives
Capers
Caesar dressing
Can also add chicken strips if desired
Combine ingredients, toss and place mixture in the center of a Low Carb Tortilla.

LOW CARB CLASSIC CLUB
Combine your favorite deli sliced meat (Roasted Turkey, Ham, Salami, or Roast Beef)
Mustard
Mayo
Lettuce
Tomatoes sliced
Italian dressing
Swiss cheese
Avocado sliced
Combine ingredients, toss and place mixture in the center of a Low Carb Tortilla.

MEDITERRANEAN WRAP
Romaine lettuce
Sun dried tomato spread
Feta cheese
Kalamatta Olives
Bermuda onions
Turkey Breast sliced or sliced green bell peppers for a vegetarian wrap
Cucumbers sliced
Combine ingredients, toss and place mixture in the center of a Low Carb Tortilla.

ROASTED & TOASTED GRILLED VEGETABLE WRAP
Grilled eggplant, bell peppers, zucchini
Wild greens
Sliced ripe tomatoes
Bermuda onion's sliced
Goat cheese
Low Carb Vinaigrette
Combine ingredients, toss and place mixture in the center of a Low Carb Tortilla.

CLASSIC BLT WRAP
Crispy bacon strips
Mayo
Lettuce
Tomato's sliced
Add sliced Turkey if desired
Combine ingredients, toss and place mixture in the center of a Low Carb Tortilla.

Gregory Pryor C.E.C.

SOUTH OF THE BORDER WRAP
Grilled steak or chicken
Lettuce
Tomatoes
Salsa
Avocado
Monterey jack cheese shredded
Fresh cilantro
Combine ingredients, toss and place mixture in the center of a Low Carb Tortilla.

ITALIAN BREAKFAST WRAP
Scramble eggs
Fresh tomatoes diced
Fresh cilantro and garlic chopped finely
Provolone cheese
Italian sausage cut up into pieces.
Combine ingredients, toss and place mixture in the center of a Low Carb Tortilla.

BREAKFAST WRAP
Scramble eggs
Diced medley of vegetables
Hot sauce
Diced ham, or bacon
Cheddar cheese
Finely chopped onions
Combine ingredients, toss and place mixture in the center of a Low Carb Tortilla

Now that we have taken a look at the possibilities and the principles of creating healthy and flavorful side dishes, I want to take a minute and recap. Let's look at where we are at this point before we get to what I consider the nucleus of the Low Carb Lifestyle, Entrée's. I hope that several of the keys to success in your new Lifestyle have become less of a mystery by now. You can see by what we've learned so far that this is not a boring complicated Lifestyle. Second, and as important to me, is that by now you recognize that your choices and recipes are those made with whole foods commonly found and what should be available in most any well stocked supermarket. With every recipe or dish I have designed it is and remains my goal to do so without you having to 1. Shop at numerous stores. 2. Buy unusual products and for the most part expensive products with again limited sources. However, most importantly to me it is my wish that from the suggestions, guidelines and directions that you will develop the thinking and creativity necessary to create many of your own recipes in a Low Carb fashion. A little later we will compare some before and after recipes, with suggestions on how you can redesign recipes to adhere to the Low Carb Lifestyle. I will show you how we spot the trouble spots within a recipe and how to reduce those to fit within your Carb Limits.

As we proceed to the many entrée recipes, let's start with breakfast. As we continue we will be using many types of cooking methods in the entrée recipes; Dry heat cooking which consist of grilling and broiling, pan frying, sautéing and roasting. We will also use moist heat cooking, which is also known as braising. This method is normally desired for less tender cuts of beef as well as for many pork, poultry and seafood items. As I present a recipe from this point on, as the recipe may require, I will offer guidelines for the style of cooking that is used.

Let's explore some breakfast ideas beyond the typical fried bacon and eggs.

BREAKFAST ENTRÉES

Egg Dishes

Baked Breakfast
Servings: 4

This dish can be assembled in many ways to create a different version to satisfy your need for variety. For example use fine diced cooked ham in place of the sausage. Another interesting example is to cut bacon slices in half and line the bottom and sides of a shallow ramekin or custard dish slightly letting the bacon lap over-the-top edge to create a "bacon basket" before adding the whole egg. You can even beat the egg and pour it in the ramekin or custard cup for a different texture and look.
I prefer to use a shallow wide custard cup or bowl, as doing so allows being able to loosen the edge of the baked egg and tilt it to slide this out on a plate for an attractive presentation.
[

4 whole eggs
4 slices bacon cooked but still pliable
1/2 pound sausage, cooked
1/2 cup cheddar cheese, grated

Preheat oven to 350°F. Spray a small ramekin or custard dish with nonstick spray. Line bottom of four muffin cups with loose sausage so it covers the bottom of each one and pat down. Wrap bacon around the inside of each cup. Crack an egg in each one. Bake approx 20 minutes until you see bacon is done. Sprinkle cheese on top of each one and bake until cheese is melted.

Nutrition per Serving
Carbs: 1 g Fiber: 0 g **Net Carbs: 1 g** Protein: 18 g Fat: 35 g Calories: 396

Gregory Pryor C.E.C.

Egg Dishes

Baked Eggs
Servings: 4

This is just another of the many variations to baked eggs. You can prepare this up to the baking stage the night before, cover with plastic wrap and store in the fridge till ready to use.

1/2 medium tomato, sliced
1/4 cup heavy cream
2 tablespoons beef stock
1 cup shredded cheddar cheese
4 whole eggs
3 sprigs fresh basil, finely chopped

Preheat oven to 325º. Grease 4 ramekins. Slice tomato and place on paper towel to absorb moisture. Beat whipping cream until it thickens slightly. Add beef stock and beat again. Place a tablespoon of cream mixture in each ramekin. Add a sprinkling of cheese and then divide the tomato slices between the ramekins. Carefully crack one egg in each ramekin. Add another tablespoon of cream and the remaining cheese. Top with fresh basil.
Bake 12-18 minutes, uncovered until eggs are set.

Nutrition per Serving
Carbs: 2 g Fiber: trace g **Net Carbs: 2 g** Protein: 13 g Fat: 19 g Calories: 236

Egg Dishes

Baked Ham and Eggs with Goat Cheese
Servings: 4

This version of Low Carb baked eggs is a true pleasure to enjoy and a real eye-opener.

3/4 cup diced cooked ham
1 10-ounce package frozen chopped spinach, thawed and drained
1/8 pound unsalted butter, melted
8 whole eggs
3 ounces goat cheese
1/2 teaspoon crushed rosemary
Salt and pepper, to taste

Preheat oven to 350º. Grease 4 individual baking dishes (large enough to hold two eggs). Divide ham into prepared dishes. Top with equal portion of spinach. Place 1 teaspoon melted butter on spinach. Carefully break 2 eggs on top of this mixture in each dish. Divide goat cheese into 4 pieces and place one-piece on top of eggs; sprinkle with rosemary, salt and pepper. Top with any remaining butter. Bake 12 - 14 minutes until eggs are set.

Nutrition per Serving
Carbs: 5 g Fiber: 2 g **Net Carbs: 3 g** Protein: 24 g Fat: 31 g Calories: 392

Gregory Pryor C.E.C.

Egg Dishes

Italian Style Frittata
Servings: 4

The many varieties of frittata's are only as limited as your imagination. Consider using sliced mushrooms, diced ham, pepperoni, shredded cheese or just about any Low Carb item that you have a taste for at the time.
Typically a frittata is considered to be an open faced omelet and is finished under a broiler to set the top. This is my preferred method; however you can cover and finished over low to medium heat, taking care not to burn the bottom.
Always if you include any meat in a frittata, just as with an omelet, use cooked meat only, well drained.

6 whole eggs
Salt and pepper, to taste
1/2 teaspoon dried sage
1/2 teaspoon dried oregano
1/2 teaspoon dried thyme
1 tablespoon butter
1 medium Roma tomato, sliced
1/3 cup fresh basil leaves, finely chopped
3 ounces cream cheese, cubed

Whisk together eggs, salt, pepper, sage, oregano and thyme. In large skillet, melt butter over medium heat. Sauté tomatoes one minute. Lower heat and add basil sautéing until wilted, 1-2 minutes. Pour egg mixture over all and top with cream cheese cubes. Cover and cook over low heat approximately 20 minutes or until set on top; or cook until bottom is partially set and finish cooking top under broiler.
Once set and firm there are several ways to serve a frittata. You can either slice the individual serving and remove with a spatula, or loosen the frittata around the edge and slide this onto a large serving plate and allow each person to serve themselves. This is an impressive presentation.

Nutrition per Serving
Carbs: 10 g Fiber: 3 g **Net Carbs: 7 g** Protein: 19 g Fat: 17 g Calories: 206

Egg Dishes

Breakfast Skillet

Servings: 1

Since nearly every breakfast menu these days offers some form of Skillet Breakfast, so shall we. Again this is but an example, feel free to use any other Low Carb additions, such as diced ham instead of sausage, crumbled crisp bacon, diced bell peppers or any other item that would be to your liking. Simply prepare this recipe or one of your own individually for each person at breakfast.

1/4 pound sausage
1/2 cup mushrooms, sliced
1/4 cup heavy cream
3 tablespoons shredded cheddar cheese
2 whole eggs

In small sauté pan add sausage, sliced mushrooms and cook, stirring often until lightly browned.
Add cream and allow to reduce by 1/3. Add cheese stir to melt.
Cook eggs however you like them and add to skillet. Gently slide onto a dinner plate.

Nutrition per Serving
Carbs: 5 g Fiber: trace g **Net Carbs: 5 g** Protein: 25 g Fat: 61 g Calories: 667

Gregory Pryor C.E.C.

Egg Dishes

Seafood Omelet
Servings: 1

Anyone having ever been to a breakfast buffet knows the varieties of omelets are endless. Any cooked meat or seafood will make a fine filling as do any combinations of sweated vegetables. Consider all the different cheeses and you can create a different type omelet for any occasion or flavor combinations.
A few things to consider when making an omelet. 1. A good nonstick omelet skillet is a necessity for cooking ease. A heat proof rubber spatula is also helpful. Never use metal with a nonstick skillet. Feeling daring? Practice flipping the omelet instead of folding. As the egg cooks lift the edges to allow uncooked egg to run under till the egg is nearly set. Loosen the edges and with a rolling motion, flip the omelet. Add your fillings and slide the omelet onto a plate folding over as it exits the pan. THIS TAKES PRACTICE, but I know you can do this, I have taught many this technique with little effort. Finally remember, classically an omelet should not be brown; it should have the same color as scrambled eggs.

1/3 cup poached salmon
OR
1/3 can salmon, drained*
1 tablespoon butter
3 eggs, beaten
1/3 tablespoon finely chopped green onion
2 tablespoons dairy sour cream
1 tablespoon finely chopped parsley
Dash salt
Dash pepper

Flake salmon. Heat 1 tablespoon butter in saucepan; add salmon and heat briefly and remove. Combine eggs, green onion, salt and pepper; mix well. Pour egg mixture into pan and cook until set. Spoon salmon over half of omelet; fold in half and turn onto warm plate. Spoon sour cream over omelet; sprinkle with parsley.

Nutrition per Serving
Carbs: 3 g Fiber: trace g **Net Carbs: 3 g** Protein: 22 g Fat: 24 g Calories: 367

Egg Dishes

Eggs Florentine
Servings: 4

A simple twist to eggs benedict. You can use a 10 ounce package of frozen spinach, squeezed dry.

2 bunches spinach, blanched
2 teaspoons shallots, finely diced
1 cup hollandaise sauce, see recipe
Salt and pepper, to taste
8 large eggs
1 cup shredded Gruyère

Sauté spinach with shallots. Add 1/2 cup sauce, salt and pepper and blend. Arrange on bottom of four serving dishes.
Poach eggs; set on top of spinach. Top each set of eggs with remaining sauce. Garnish with shredded Gruyère cheese.

Nutrition per Serving
Carbs: 7 g Fiber: 2 g **Net Carbs: 5 g** Protein: 21 g Fat: 48 g Calories: 580

TIPS FOR POACHING EGGS.

For eggs to hold their shape when poached, they should be fresh. A solid, firm white will prevent the yolk from breaking. A little vinegar (2 tablespoons per quart) in the cooking water will help coagulate egg whites and keep poached eggs from spreading as they cook.

Poach eggs in part water, part broth for added flavor. Bring the poaching liquid to a boil, and then reduce to a simmer before adding eggs.

Crack cold eggs, one at a time, into a saucer or custard cup. Holding the dish close to the liquid's surface, gently slip each egg into the simmering liquid. If you're not using egg rings, use a spoon to corral the egg white and pull it toward the yolk.

A poached egg won't spread as much if you use a spoon to form a whirlpool in the poaching water and then slide the egg into the vortex.

Test for doneness by using a slotted spoon to lift each egg from the water; press with your fingertip. The white should be firm, the yolk soft.

Drain poached eggs briefly on paper towels to remove excess liquid.

Poached eggs can be made in advance and stored until you're ready to use them. Have a bowl of ice water standing by; plunge the cooked eggs directly into the cold water. Cover and refrigerate for up to 2 days.

To reheat poached eggs that have been made in advance, use a slotted spoon to set them in hot water for a minute, or just until warmed through.

Egg Dishes

Eggs Benedict
Servings: 2

Use a large round cutter to cut approx a 3 to 3 1/2 inch circle from each slice of Low Carb Bread. The net grams for each circle is less than the 4g for entire slice.
Slice either a square or diamond shape from black olive for garnish. Sprinkle with parsley.

4 whole poached egg
2 slices Canadian bacon, or ham
2 slices Nature Own Low Carb Bread, see notes
Hollandaise Sauce
Chopped parsley
Sliced black olive for garnish

Melt 1-2 Tb butter in a small frying pan and cook the Canadian bacon or ham slices until lightly browned. Toast the bread rounds and butter them while warm. Poach the eggs as described. Place one bread round on each plate, add a slice of ham and two poached eggs. Top with hollandaise and garnish with an olive garnish as noted and chopped parsley.

Nutrition per Serving
Carbs: 6 g Fiber: 1 g **Net Carbs: 5 g** Protein: 18 g Fat: 12 g Calories: 194

Egg Dishes

Scrambled Eggs and Lox
Servings: 4

There is a trick to making "scrambled eggs" and "great scrambled eggs"
The first is never use high heat. Second to make "great scrambled eggs'
always continue to stir and move the eggs. Those typical flat dry scrambled
eggs many of us have had were a result of letting the eggs sit and barley
stirring the eggs during cooking. Finally I always add for every two eggs
approx 1 tablespoon of cream cheese into the pan at the same time as the
eggs. This will melt into the eggs adding flavor, moisture and body to the
eggs.
No matter what other versions of scrambled eggs you like, rather it be plain,
with diced ham, sausage, diced vegetables, the cooking principle is the
same.

12 whole eggs, beaten
Salt and pepper, to taste
8 ounces cream cheese cut in 1" cubes
2 tablespoons butter
6 ounces lox, chopped

Whisk eggs, salt and pepper in large bowl to blend.
Melt butter in large nonstick skillet over medium-high heat.
Add eggs and cream cheese. Using a wooden spoon, stir until eggs are
almost set, about 5 minutes. Gently add salmon and stir just until eggs are
set, about 1-minute.
Transfer eggs to platter. Sprinkle with chives, if desired, and serve.

Nutrition per Serving
Carbs: 3 g Fiber: 0 g **Net Carbs: 3 g** Protein: 29 g Fat: 41 g Calories: 495

Breakfast

Crepes and Fruit

Servings: 4

Want something sweet for breakfast, here it is. I use a crepe' pan for the crepe's, however a small nonstick pan will serve the same task.

3 whole eggs, beaten
3 tablespoons all-purpose flour
1/4 teaspoon salt
1/3 cup heavy cream
3/4 cup ricotta cheese
1/4 cup steels fruit filling
1 tablespoon Splenda®
1 1/2 tablespoons butter

In a medium bowl, whisk eggs, flour and salt until smooth. Gradually whisk in cream. Let stand 5 minutes. Batter should be thin enough to spread evenly in the bottom of the pan.
Press ricotta through a fine sieve into a small bowl. Mix in fruit spread and Splenda®.
Melt butter in a small nonstick skillet over medium heat. Pour in 2 tablespoons batter and tilt pan coat bottom.
Cook until golden on bottom; turn over. Cook 1-minute more. Transfer to a plate. Repeat with remaining batter. Spread pancakes with ricotta mixture and roll up.

Nutrition per Serving
Carbs: 7 g Fiber: 1 g **Net Carbs: 6 g** Protein: 10 g Fat: 21 g Calories: 257

Breakfast

Waffle

Servings: 4

This recipe was a huge success at a Low Carb Show that I attended and served many Low Carb specialties, some of which you will find in this book. Few if any that sampled this could believe it was anything less than the traditional waffle.

There is a trick here. After you cook the waffle in the waffle iron (I prefer the Belgium style) let the waffle cool. If you're going to use these right away, after the waffle cools, reheat till crisp in a 400 degree oven on a cookie sheet. This crisps them nicely. If they fit in your toaster this works fine as well. These freeze perfectly, so make ahead of time, freeze and toast when needed. Served with either Carb Free or reduced carb syrup or steels fruit makes a wonderful breakfast.

The batter will be a bit thick which is how it needs to be. You may have to adjust the consistency a bit, if so add a few drops of water. The batter should not run on the waffle maker, but instead have to be spread over the surface.

This sometimes takes a little practice to get the batter just right for your waffle iron, but with a little practice you will be making these by the dozens to freeze.

3 whole large eggs
1/4 cup heavy cream
1/4 cup sour cream
2 tablespoons butter, melted
2 tablespoons Splenda®
1/4 cup soy flour
1/2 teaspoon baking powder
1 teaspoon vanilla extract, or to taste

In blender, mix first four ingredients and blend until creamy. Add dry ingredients; blend until well mixed and creamy. Spray your waffle maker with Pam. Prepare as usual for your waffle maker.

Nutrition per Serving
Carbs: 4 g Fiber: 1 g **Net Carbs: 3 g** Protein: 7 g Fat: 19 g Calories: 215

Now having reviewed these recipes you can see the choices and varieties are nearly endless. I will emphasis the most logical choice for breakfast when following the Low Carb Lifestyle is one consisting of breakfast meat and eggs, why? To prevent those false cravings for more sweets throughout the day, and more importantly to keep the fat burning metabolism this Lifestyle supports. It has been my experience to always start my day with a greater fat and protein content for just that reason, plus I prefer to save my personal allowed Carbs for later in the day at dinner or for that rich piece of cheesecake with fruit when that desire overcomes me. There is one commonly agreed on fact shared throughout the people in the *"know"* involved in the study of the success of the Low Carb Lifestyle. The fewer Carbs from sugar and starch, the more successful the results. And those results can be measured in several ways, such as, weight loss, fat loss resulting in smaller body mass, greater levels of energy and above all a greater enjoyment of life. Again as we review the following recipes I want to emphasis again, the wish I have to provide you with wholesome, flavorful and whole food recipes that easily will satisfy the guidelines for a Low Carb Lifestyle.

We are going to explore the largest selections and varieties of recipes we can enjoy on our Low Carb Lifestyle. The main course entrées that we will prepare can and will vary from simple to complex, but as before I encourage you to experiment with these more complex recipes. The reward is well worth the added time and effort. In truth even the more complex recipes are not that difficult if as we talked about before you are properly organized and fully prepared. Before you begin any recipe take some time to familiarize yourself with it, make certain you have all the needed ingredients and cookware. And remember most of all, this is just cooking, it is not rocket science. Since many of the following recipes will require Ghee or Clarified Butter, let me take this time to explain how to make this product. I make five pounds at a time, as I use this for nearly every aspect of cooking daily, from simple fried eggs, omelets, sautéing and for basting many baked items. The amount you make depends entirely just how much you will use in a weeks time. It keeps just fine covered and stored in the fridge.

Clarified Butter or *Ghee*, also sometimes called **drawn butter**, is regular butter that has been treated to remove any nonfat elements to improve its qualities as a cooking medium. Butter has two main parts: butterfat and milk proteins; there's also a lot of water, sometimes up to 18 percent. Salted butter of course contains salt, too; for clarified butter, use only unsalted, as salt can lower the smoking point of the finished product and defeat the purpose of clarifying.

Without the milk proteins, clarified butter can be heated to higher temperatures without forming brown specks or eventually burning, so it's good for gentle sautéing, or for more vigorous frying when mixed with a little olive or vegetable oil to boost its smoking point.

The standard method for making clarified butter is to melt the butter gently in a sturdy saucepan until you see the butterfat separating and forming a thick layer in the pan. Most of the milk solids will drop to the bottom of the pan, and a layer of white foam will form on top. Remove the pan from the heat gently, so you don't disturb the layers, spoon off the top layer of foam, and carefully pour off the pure butterfat into a clean container. Discard the milky residue from the bottom of the pan.

Another method is to melt the butter and then boil it until the milk solids set and clump together at the bottom of the pan and the butterfat floats on top. If this method is taken further to the point where the milk proteins harden and darken slightly, the butterfat intensifies in flavor and color and is known as *ghee,* which is a mainstay of Indian cooking. The smoking point of ghee is slightly higher than that of regular clarified butter. Again, carefully decant the clarified butter and discard the milky leftovers, or strain it through a sieve lined with paper towel or cheesecloth.

Once you've made clarified butter, you can store it in the refrigerator for several weeks, but be sure to keep it covered because fat absorbs odors easily. Use it for sautéing, for flavoring cake, yes I said cake, we will make several cakes later that we can flavor with this butter or crepe batters, for tossing with steamed vegetables, or for brushing on a piece of poached fish for moisture and flavor.

MAIN DISH ENTRÉE'S

So many of the recipes that I will include on the following pages are but a small sampling of the overall number of variations to your meal plans available. Apart from the obvious and many choices such as fired or grilled hamburgers, basic grilled or broiled steaks. What makes a great burger "*GREAT*"? Here are my thoughts

What makes a great hamburger? First, there's the meat. You want to use a flavorful cut, like sirloin, chuck or round if you are feeding a large group on a budget. The meat should be ground twice, first through the course plate of the grinder, then through the fine plate, and it shouldn't be too lean. Fifteen to twenty percent of fat is ideal.

I adhere to the "*less is more*" school when it comes to making hamburgers. Namely, the fewer ingredients you add to the meat, the better. Oh, I know how tempting it is for cooks to want to season the meat with onion, garlic, spices and condiments, but to taste a burger at its best, keep it pure and simple. The garnishes will add all the flavor you need.

One final bit of advice: handle the meat as little as possible; anything more will rob the burger of its juiciness and primal flavor.

179

Gregory Pryor C.E.C.

INGREDIENTS FOR BURGERS:

2 pounds ground round, chuck or sirloin

2 tablespoons unsalted butter, melted or olive oil

Salt and freshly ground black pepper to taste

6 slices (½-inch thick) Vidalia onion or other sweet onion (optional)

INGREDIENTS FOR THE TOPPINGS: (ANY OR ALL)

Iceberg lettuce leaves

Sliced, fresh, ripe tomatoes

Sliced dill or sweet pickles No sugar added

Cooked bacon, 2 strips per burger

Cheese Slices

Low Carb ketchup

Mustard

Mayonnaise

Preheat the grill to high. Divide meat into 6 equal portions. Lightly wet your hands with cold water, and then form each portion of meat into a round patty, 4 inches across and of even thickness. When ready to cook, oil the grill grate. Brush 1 side of the patties and the onion slices lightly with melted butter and season with salt and pepper. Arrange both the burgers and onion slices butter side down on the hot grate and grill until nicely browned, about 4 minutes. Brush the other side lightly with more melted butter and season with more salt and pepper. Turn with a spatula and continue grilling until nicely browned and cooked to taste, about 4 minutes for medium. Alternately if grilling is not a choice, you can pan fry these same burgers in a large skillet over medium heat. Set out toppings.

I will give you several versions of these simple items with variations. I will share with you several different Low Carb Fried Chicken recipes as well as Low Carb Meat Loaf with gravy. I will share with you many classical recipes, many of which can be changed by simply selecting a different meat item, and prepared in much the same way. For example; Veal Piccata, just as easily could be Chicken Piccata, Pork Piccata or Turkey Piccata. Again another example would be Veal Parmigiana; here Chicken is often used in the same manner. Fish is another example of how we can vary a recipe just simply by using a different fresh fish. Several years ago when Blackened Red Fish appeared on many menus, few if anyone then even considered that this same style of preparation would and did apply to so many other available fresh fish choices. Nowadays we see nearly every fish offered blackened, many such others as, grouper, dolphin, Sea bass, snapper, catfish and even shrimp. More and more we see these same seafood items offered grilled. Grilled fish when properly cooked is one great pleasure from the sea. Think about grilled swordfish, with any of the many sides we talked about and a simple tossed salad, now there is a complete meal. Remember early on in the book when I said to you that many of the classical recipes from many years ago are by design Low in Carbs. Well now I will prove my point in the many classical recipes I will provide to you on the following pages. One final note, always look for the freshest quality products available, as I have said time and again, always use the finest products available, there is no substitution for quality.

BEEF

Grilled Steak Guidelines

1. Meat should always be at room temperature before it is cooked. Remove your steaks from the refrigerator at least half an hour before you are ready to cook.
2. Preheat broiler or grill to maximum temperature.
3. Rub both sides of the steaks with coarse or kosher salt and pepper.
4. Place the steaks 3 to 5 inches from the flame to sear the outside and seal in the juices. *(To check temperature, cautiously hold hand about 4 inches above coals. Medium coals will force removal of hand in 4 seconds)*.
5. Turn the steaks after 2 to 3 minutes.
6. After the steaks have been seared on both sides, remove from heat, and brush both sides with extra virgin olive oil. This will help form the crust that adds the touch of perfection.
7. Return the steaks to heat and cook on both sides to a desired doneness.
8. Transfer to warmed dinner plates or a platter, and let rest five minutes before serving.

Approximate total cooking times are listed below for a preheated oven broiler. Red-hot charcoal may take less time. Give filet mignon one minute less to cook than other steaks. *DO NOT OVERCOOK*

This table represents *total* cooking times

Cooking Times			
Thickness	1 inch	1-1/4 inches	1-3/4 inches
Rare	10 minutes	12 minutes	15 minutes
Medium	15 minutes	17 minutes	20 minutes
Medium Well	20 minutes	22 minutes	25 minutes

Entrées & Main Dishes, Beef

Basic Low Carb Meat loaf Mixture

Although this formula or mixture seems like a large amount it is simple to make the meatloaves ahead of time and freeze till ready to use. What I like to do is make up a batch of this mixture and fill bread loaf pans, wrap and freeze. Here is where I again use my vacuum packaging system. Another smart example is you may also fill individual size loaf pans and freeze as well for just as many individual size meatloaves as you may need on any given day. Just remember to take these out the night before and allow to thaw in the fridge. The convenience of having this made ahead of time and ready for use is worth the volume you produce with this recipe. The net Carbs per serving based on an 8 ounce portion of this mixture is 4g.

6 pounds ground chuck
4 pounds lean ground pork
3 cups finely diced onions sweated
2 cups finely diced celery sweated
1/4 cup diced garlic (optional)
1 cup finely sliced green onions
1 cup chopped parsley
6 whole eggs
1 cup heavy whipping cream
Salt and cracked pepper to taste

In a large mixing bowl, combine ground chuck, pork, onions, celery, garlic, green onions and parsley. Using your hands, mix the ingredients thoroughly until all seasonings are well blended. Add eggs, whipping cream, salt and pepper. Continue to blend until the liquids are well incorporated. Divide mixture into desired portions for later use. Freeze up to three months. To defrost, place in refrigerator overnight. Alternately you may shape and cook this mixture as you would normally, however the frozen in the pan saves muss and fuss when in a hurry. Top with Low Carb Ketchup or Chimichurri sauce for a real zest of flavor.

Entrées & Main Dishes, Beef

Blue Cheese Fillet of Beef

Servings: 4

The fillet should be about 8 ounces. You may also substitute any good cut of beef such as, 10 ounce strip steak, rib steak or sirloin. Take care to buy a good quality cut of beef as we described in the beef section in this book.

4 beef tenderloin steaks
1 large clove garlic, halved
2 teaspoons chopped fresh parsley
CHEESE TOPPING
2 tablespoons cream cheese, softened
4 teaspoons crumbled blue cheese
4 teaspoons sour cream
2 teaspoons minced onion
Dash white pepper

In small bowl, combine topping ingredients and reserve.
Rub each side of beefsteaks with garlic. Place steaks on rack in broiler pan so surface of meat is 2 to 3 inches from heat. Broil 5 to 6 minutes. Season with 1/4 teaspoon salt. Turn and broil 5 to 6 minutes. Season with an additional 1/4 teaspoon salt. Top each steak with an equal amount of reserved cheese topping. Broil an another 1 to 2 minutes. Garnish with parsley.

Nutrition per Serving
Carbs: 1 g Fiber: 0 g **Net Carbs: 1 g** Protein: 19 g Fat: 27 g Calories: 328

Entrées & Main Dishes, Beef

Grilled Herb Steaks
Servings: 2

2 well-trimmed boneless beef top loin or rib eye steaks, cut 1 inch thick (roughly 1 pound)
Salt
HERB MUSTARD
2 large cloves garlic, crushed
2 teaspoons water
2 tablespoons Dijon-style mustard
1 teaspoon dried basil leaves
1/2 teaspoon pepper
1/2 teaspoon dried thyme leaves

Stir together mustard ingredients; spread onto both sides of beefsteaks.
Place steaks on grille over medium, ash-covered coals. Grill top loin steaks, uncovered, 15 to 18 minutes (rib eye steaks 11 to 14 minutes) for medium rare to medium doneness, turning occasionally. Season steaks with salt, as desired. Serve whole or carve steaks crosswise into thick slices.

Nutrition per Serving
Carbs: 1 g Fiber: 0 g **Net Carbs: 1 g** Protein: 25 g Fat: 7 g Calories: 171

Entrées & Main Dishes, Veal

Classic Veal Osso Buco
Servings: 4

Have your butcher cut the veal Osso Buco from the desirable hind shank into hefty 2 1/2-inch sections. If your butcher didn't already tie these for you be certain to ask him to do so. Your finished dish will be tender, succulent and juicy.

This is another example of using two cooking methods; however the main and most important is the slow simmer, or braising. Be certain to get an even dark brown color when browning the veal.

4 large veal shanks see notes
3 tablespoons clarified butter
2 tablespoons olive oil
1 medium carrot, minced
1 medium onion, minced
1 stalk celery, chopped
1/2 cup dry white wine
1 cup brown stock
2 medium tomatoes, peeled seeded and chopped
Salt and pepper, to taste
GREMOLATA GARNISH
1/2 Cup parsley, minced fine
2 teaspoons lemon zest, minced
2 cloves garlic, minced

Select a heavy-bottomed pot with a cover, just large enough to hold the veal shanks in one layer. Combine the butter and the oil in the pot and heat until hot but not smoking. Add the veal and brown well on all sides over moderate heat.

Transfer the veal to a platter. Add the vegetables to the pot, and cook until just softened, about 5 minutes.

Return the veal to the pot and add the white wine, the stock and the tomatoes. Season to taste with salt and pepper. Cover the pot and bring to a boil, and then turn heat to low. Simmer gently for about 1 1/2 hours, turning the meat occasionally, and adding a little extra stock to the pot if necessary. The Osso Buco is done when the meat is tender, and the sauce is slightly thickened. Transfer the Osso Buco to a platter and keep warm.

Prepare the gremolata. Combine the parsley, lemon zest and garlic in a small bowl. Season to taste with salt and pepper. Sprinkle the gremolata over the Osso Buco and serve on warm dinner plates.

Nutrition per Serving
Carbs: 9 g Fiber: 2 g **Net Carbs: 7 g** Protein: 1 g Fat: 17 g Calories: 202

Entrées & Main Dishes, Veal

Sauté of Veal Medallions
Servings: 4

I think you will find this to be as simple a recipe to prepare as any in this book, but don't let the simple fool you; this is one robustly flavored dish. Tender veal and the rich brown stock combine to reward the palette. When I am in a rush, this recipe served with mock horseradish smashers and sautéed Swiss chard make a rich rewarding meal. This is an example of why I strongly urge you to make your own brown stock; the reduction in the pan of this rich stock is the reason for the wonderful flavor the sauce builds on top of the veal.

8 small veal medallions, about 3 oz. each
Salt and pepper, to taste
2 tablespoons clarified butter
4 medium button mushrooms, quartered
1/2 cup brown stock
1 tablespoon cold butter

Pat the veal medallions dry with paper towels. Season both sides with salt and pepper.
Heat the butter in a large sauté pan over medium-high heat. Sauté the veal medallions until golden, about 2 minutes per side. Do not crowd the pan-sauté in batches if necessary so the medallions brown properly.
Remove finished medallions to a platter and keep warm in a 180° F oven.
Add the mushrooms to the pan and sauté briefly till slightly browned. Add the stock to the sauté pan, and increase heat to high. Bring to a boil and stir for 2 minutes, until the sauce is slightly thickened. Remove from the heat and add the cold butter, swirl the pan to blend. Spoon the finished sauce over the medallions and serve.

Nutrition per Serving
Carbs: 3 g Fiber: 1 g **Net Carbs: 2 g** Protein: 1 g Fat: 9 g Calories: 98

Gregory Pryor C.E.C.

Entrées & Main Dishes, Veal

Roasted Veal Breast
Servings: 4-6

1 veal breast
1 clove garlic
Salt and pepper
Paprika
4 onions
2 cups brown stock

Take 1 meaty veal breast. Rub it with a cut clove of garlic. Season with salt, pepper and paprika. Place in shallow roasting pan. Place 4 onions peeled and cut in half around the roast. Pour in 2 cups brown stock. Bake at 400° for 1/2 hr. Turn heat to 350° and bake another hour, or until tender. Remove meat and onions. Place baking pan over low heat on top stove. Heat the sauce, loosening brown bits in pan. Add more stock if necessary. Simmer till slightly thickened. Season to taste. Serve with veal.

Nutrition per Serving
Carbs: 6 g Fiber: 1 g **Net Carbs: 5 g** Protein: 2 g Fat: trace g Calories: 34

Entrées & Main Dishes, Beef

Teriyaki Grilled Steak

Servings: 6

Tip: Beef can be marinated in a plastic bag, glass utility dish or other nonreactive container. Acidic ingredients and alcohol react with some metals, such as aluminum and iron, to discolor food and pass on a metallic flavor.
Choose a container in which the beef fits snugly and lies flat.

1 (2 pound) well-trimmed beef top round or sirloin steak, cut 1-1/2 inches thick
MARINADE
3/4 cup teriyaki sauce
2 tablespoons dry white wine
1 tablespoon finely chopped fresh ginger

In small bowl, combine marinade ingredients; mix well. Place steak and marinade in plastic bag, turning to coat.
Close bag securely and marinate in refrigerator 6 to 8 hours (or overnight, if desired), turning occasionally.
Remove steak from marinade; discard marinade. Place steak on grill over medium, ash-covered coals; grill, 25 to 28 minutes for medium rare doneness, turning occasionally.
Carve steak crosswise into thin slices.

Nutrition per Serving
Carbs: 2 g Fiber: 0 g **Net Carbs: 2 g** Protein: 33 g Fat: 3 g Calories: 198

Entrées & Main Dishes, Beef

Savory Mushroom-Stuffed Steak

Servings: 4

A boneless beef top sirloin steak will yield four 3-ounce cooked, trimmed servings per pound.

3 pound beef top sirloin steak, boneless
1 tablespoon olive oil
1 cup fresh mushrooms, finely chopped
1/4 cup minced shallots
OR
1/4 cup minced green onions
1 tablespoon dry red wine
1/4 teaspoon salt
1/4 teaspoon dried thyme
1/4 teaspoon pepper

Heat oil in heavy nonstick skillet over medium-high heat. Add mushrooms and shallots; cook 4 to 5 minutes or until vegetables are tender, stirring occasionally. Add wine and cook until evaporated. Stir in salt, thyme and pepper.
Remove from heat; cool thoroughly. Meanwhile trim excess fat from beef top sirloin steak. To cut pocket in steak, make horizontal cut through center of steak, parallel to surface of meat, about 1 inch from each side. Cut to, but not through, opposite side. Spoon cooled stuffing into pocket, spreading evenly. Secure opening with wooden picks. Place steak on rack in broiler pan so surface of meat is 4 to 5 inches from heat. Broil 26 to 32 minutes for rare to medium, turning once. Place on warm serving platter. Cover with aluminum foil tent and allow to rest 10 to 15 minutes. Remove wooden picks. Trim excess fat from steak; carve steak into 1/2-inch thick slices.

Nutrition per Serving
Carbs: 1 g Fiber: 0 g **Net Carbs: 1 g** Protein: 62 g Fat: 52 g Calories: 741

Entrées & Main Dishes, Beef

Mexican Flank Steak and Mock Tamales
Servings: 6

To check temperature, cautiously hold hand about 4 inches above coals. Medium coals will force removal of hand in 4 seconds.

1 1/2 pounds beef flank steak, well-trimmed
1/3 cup fresh lemon juice
1/3 cup extravirgin olive oil
6 tablespoons jalapeño peppers, minced
1 tablespoon fresh cilantro, minced
1 teaspoon salt
1 teaspoon black pepper, freshly ground
Chimichurri Sauce, see recipe
Mock Tamales, see recipe optional
Lemon slices
Jalapeño peppers
Cilantro sprigs

Combine lemon juice, oil, jalapeño peppers, cilantro, salt and black pepper. Reserve 1/4 cup marinade. Place beef flank steak in plastic bag; add remaining marinade, turning to coat. Close bag securely and marinate in refrigerator 6 to 8 hours (or overnight, if desired), turning occasionally. Prepare Chimichurri Sauce. About 15 minutes before grilling, prepare Mock Tamales. Remove steak from marinade; discard marinade. Place steak on grid over medium coals (see notes). Place mock tamales around outer edge of grill. Grill steak and mock tamales 12 to 15 minutes for rare to medium, turning steak and tamales once and brushing steak occasionally with reserved marinade. Place steak and tamales on warm platter. Spoon 1/4 cup of Chimichurri Sauce over tamales. Garnish platter with lemon slices, jalapeño peppers and cilantro sprigs. Carve steak diagonally across the grain into thin slices. Serving Ideas: Serve steak and tamales with remaining salsa.

Nutrition per Serving
Carbs: 4 g Fiber: 1 g **Net Carbs: 3 g** Protein: 23 g Fat: 24 g Calories: 333

Gregory Pryor C.E.C.

DIPS/SALSA, SAUCES

Chimichurri Sauce
Servings: 6

Here is another of those sauces that one can alter in many ways to adapt flavors or needs. I enjoy this as a spicy sauce for fish. Replace one fresh jalapeño pepper with either a half or whole depending on heat, chipotle pepper finely chopped and 1/2 teaspoon of the adobo sauce. This makes a wonderful zesty red sauce. Be certain to use caution when using these fiery peppers.

1 cup parsley, flat leaf
6 cloves garlic, peeled
2 jalapeno peppers, seeded
5 tablespoons extra virgin olive oil
3 tablespoons red wine vinegar
1 teaspoon kosher salt
1/4 teaspoon old bay Seafood seasoning

In a food processor, combine parsley, garlic and jalapenos; process until a chunky paste forms. Drizzle in oil while pulsing processor, stir in vinegar and season to taste with salt.

Nutrition per Serving
Carbs: 2 g Fiber: 1 g **Net Carbs: 1 g** Protein: 1 g Fat: 11 g Calories: 110

Miscellaneous

Mock Tamales

Servings: 6
Preparation Time: 15 minutes
1 cup sharp Cheddar cheese, shredded
1 cup Muenster cheese, shredded
2 tablespoons minced green onions with tops
6 Low Carb tortillas

Combine Cheddar cheese, Muenster cheese and green onions. Place equal amounts of cheese mixture in center of each tortilla. Fold bottom side of tortilla over filling; fold two sides in over filling. Fold down topside of tortilla enclosing filling. Wrap each mock tamale in 8 × 12-inch sheet of aluminum foil, twisting each end.

Nutrition per Serving
Carbs: 5 g Fiber: 1 g **Net Carbs: 4 g** Protein: 12 g Fat: 14 g Calories: 250

Entrées & Main Dishes, Beef

Chateaubriand Roast with Mushroom Sauce

Servings: 4

A luxurious and elegant roast. Cut from the center of the tenderloin filet, the Chateaubriand can be the centerpiece in a cozy dinner for two, while the Chateau roast can highlight a chic dinner for four. Choose the larger Tenderloin roast for six people.

This is often prepared and served table side in better restaurants. It can serve with any number of rich sauces made from brown stock. In this case I will suggest a simple mushroom and red wine sauce, where simple reduction is the key to a smooth rich sauce.

Ask your butcher for exactly what size roast you need for the number of servings you will be preparing. When serving this, slice the roast in 1/2 to 3/4 inch slices, shingle these on the plate and spoon the sauce over the slices, garnish with fine chopped parsley for an eye appealing presentation to match the rich flavor of this dish.

Always allow any meat item to rest before cutting. The resting time allows the juices in the meat to reabsorb and create better moisture and flavor. Resting times will vary on the size of the item, from 5 minutes for a steak, to 30 minutes for a larger roast. Allow one of this size to rest covered for 10 minutes.

1 whole chateaubriand, about 2 pounds, at room temperature
1 tablespoon extra virgin olive oil
1 tablespoon coarse salt
1 tablespoon black pepper

Preheat oven to 425 F. Dry the roast on paper towels. Rub the roast all over with olive oil, and season generously with coarse salt and freshly ground pepper. Roast for about 25 minutes for medium rare.

Remove from oven and let rest for 10 minutes before carving. Transfer to a warmed serving platter. Serve with Mushroom or Bordelaise Sauce.

Nutrition per Serving
Carbs: 1 g Fiber: 0 g **Net Carbs: 1 g** Protein: 2 g Fat: 3 g Calories: 234

Sauces

Mushroom Sauce
Servings: 4

The simple key to this sauce is the reduction. As the brown stock reduces it with thicken and intensify in flavor. You choose any shape mushroom that pleases you, sliced, halved, or quartered.

2 tablespoons clarified butter
1 whole shallot, minced
1 clove garlic, minced fine (optional)
1/2 cup mushrooms
1 cup brown stock
1/4 cup dry red wine
1 tablespoon cold butter

Melt the butter in a heavy skillet and sauté the shallot until transparent.
Add garlic and sauté 1-minute, do not brown garlic. Add the mushrooms and sauté just till the mushroom begin to give off their liquid. Add the brown stock and red wine and bring to a simmer and allow to reduce by 1/3 or until slightly thickened. Remove from the heat and add cold butter, swirl the pan to blend. Serve hot.

Nutrition per Serving
Carbs: 1 g Fiber: 0 g **Net Carbs: 1 g** Protein: trace g Fat: 9 g Calories: 97

Gregory Pryor C.E.C.

Beef, Entrées & Main Dishes

Bourbon Steak
Servings: 1

This recipe is especially useful for larger and less tender cuts of beef. This works equally well for those better more tender cuts as well. I offered this as a special many times in the Country Club as Jack Daniels Steak which was always popular.
The bourbon is a good natural tenderizer for the beef. A logical choice would be a center cut strip steak; however sirloin, rib eye or filet works just as well.
I would serve this steak with any of the mushroom side dishes listed in the book with mock horseradish smashers.

10 ounces steak, see notes
1 teaspoon Splenda®
1/4 cup bourbon
2 tablespoons soy sauce
2 tablespoons water
1 clove garlic, crushed

Mix all ingredients together, place in zip lock bag and marinate steak 4 hours or overnight.
Grill to desired doneness.

Nutrition per Serving
Carbs: 1 g Fiber: 0 g **Net Carbs: 1 g** Protein: 41 g Fat: 50 g Calories: 627

Entrées & Main Dishes, Beef

Standing Rib Roast

Servings: 4

The most desirable of all beef roasts. Traditional choices for festive occasions, these tender roasts are impressive in presentation and a delight on the palate, exquisitely flavorful and tender. Choose a roast with the bone for enriched flavor and mouthwatering appeal. Or select a boneless roast for easier carving and serving.

There are several ways to buy this roast, choose the one that better serves your needs. You can choose "on the bone oven ready" but make certain the chine bone is removed for easy carving. Or you can choose to have the roast cut from the bone and tied back on, simply ask that your butcher do this for you. The nice part of this style is the better flavor of cooking the roast on the bone and the ease of cutting the string and removing the bone(s) before carving. Finally you can buy "boneless oven ready" No matter your choice simply follow the steps here for a delicious roast.

This roast should rest at least 15 minutes before carving. This particular roast doesn't require but a simple seasoning of coarse salt and pepper. However should you like to add other flavors such as garlic, and herbs feel free to do so. For my choice I enjoy simple is best for this roast.

1 prime rib, 3 1/2 to 4 pounds
2 tablespoons olive oil
Coarse salt and pepper, as needed

Preheat your oven to 400 degrees.
Rub the olive oil over the entire roast and season well with salt and pepper.
Place the roast either on a broiler rack or a screen rack over a large baking sheet pan.
Transfer the roast, bone side down, or if boneless fat side up to the oven. After 15 minutes reduce the oven to 325 and continue to cook for approx. For 1-hour and 20 minutes to 1-hour and 30 minutes for rare, or longer for more well done meat. After 1-hour, insert an instant-read thermometer in the thickest part of the meat (not too close to the bone). When the thermometer registers 130 F (for rare meat) to 140 F (for medium-rare meat), remove the roast from the grill and let rest for 15 minutes before carving. Do not overcook. Serve with horseradish cream sauce.

Nutrition per Serving
Carbs: 1 g Fiber: 0 g **Net Carbs: 1 g** Protein: 1 g Fat: 9 g Calories: 81

Gregory Pryor C.E.C.

Sauces

Horseradish Cream Sauce
Servings: 4

1/4 cup sour cream
1/4 cup mayonnaise
2 tablespoons prepared horseradish, or to taste
1 teaspoon salt

In a mixing bowl combine all ingredients. Taste and adjust the horseradish to your own taste.

Nutrition per Serving
Carbs: 1 g Fiber: 0 g **Net Carbs: 1 g** Protein: 1 g Fat: 15 g Calories: 133

Entrées & Main Dishes, Beef

Open-Faced Steak Sandwich
Servings: 1

Always choose a well marbled minute steak. The various cuts from which these are cut from can make a difference in tough to tender. Ask your butcher for one cut from either the strip, rib or shell roast.

1/2 small red onion, sliced thin
2 tablespoons olive oil
1 tablespoon fresh rosemary, chopped
1 minute steak approx. 6 oz.
1 tablespoon Dijon-style mustard
1 tablespoon mayonnaise
1 slice tomato, ripe
1 tablespoon blue cheese, crumbled
Salt and pepper, to taste

Combine the red onion with the olive oil and the chopped rosemary. Let marinate for 1-hour, or as long as 12 hours.
Season the steak and grill or broil the minute steak just until rare. Remove from grill or broiler, to a warm plate and let rest for five minutes.
Prepare the sandwich. Spread mayonnaise and Dijon mustard to taste on the steak. Spoon any accumulated juices from the plate over the steak. Top with the tomato slice. Finish the sandwich by spooning some of the red onion mixture over the steak, followed by the Blue cheese.

Nutrition per Serving
Carbs: 4 g Fiber: 3 g **Net Carbs: 1 g** Protein: 25 g Fat: 56g Calories: 9643

Entrées & Main Dishes, Beef

Skillet Tournedos of Beef

Servings: 2

4 fillet mignons, 3 oz. each
1/4 cup clarified butter
1/4 cup shallots, diced
1/4 cup green onion, sliced
1/2 cup mushroom, sliced
1/4 cup dry red wine
2 cups brown stock
Salt and pepper, to taste

In a heavy-bottom sauté pan, melt butter over medium-high heat. Season medallions lightly with salt and pepper. Sauté in butter until golden-brown on each side, but do not burn.

Move the medallions over to one side of the skillet then add shallots, garlic, green onions and mushrooms. Sauté 2-3 minutes or until vegetables are wilted. Add red wine to deglaze pan and reduce to 1/4 cup. Add brown stock, bring to a rolling boil and reduce to about 1 cup, turning beef occasionally. Season sauce with salt and pepper.

Nutrition per Serving
Carbs: 6 g Fiber: 1 g **Net Carbs: 5 g** Protein: 36 g Fat: 71 g Calories: 829

Entrées & Main Dishes, Beef

Braised Beef Short Ribs
Servings: 4

As we talked about before braising is a method used on tougher cuts of meat that guarantees tenderness. In addition, this slow-cooked method imparts a wonderful flavor because of the longer cooking time with vegetables, herbs and stock. Beef ribs are one of many examples where we will use the braising method to create a dish.

4 pounds beef short ribs
6 slices bacon, chopped
1 large onion, quartered
2 stalks celery, chopped
3 cups brown stock
1/2 cup dry red wine
3 sprigs fresh thyme
2 sprigs fresh rosemary
6 sprigs fresh basil leaf
Salt and pepper, to taste

Preheat oven to 375 degrees F. Season short ribs well using salt and pepper. In a 10-quart Dutch oven, brown bacon to render fat over medium-high heat. Do not burn. Remove crisp bacon and set aside. In the bacon fat brown short ribs, 4 at a time, taking care not to burn bacon fat. Once all the ribs are brown add onions and celery. Sauté 2-3 minutes to tenderize vegetables. Add brown stock and red wine. Bring to a rolling boil and reduce to simmer. Add cooked bacon, browned short ribs, thyme, rosemary and basil. Season stock with additional salt and pepper if necessary. Return the mixture to a rolling boil, cover and place in preheated oven. Cook 1 ½ hours, checking for tenderness. When ribs are fork-tender, remove from stock and set aside. Reduce stock by half.
When ready to serve, strain stock, return ribs to the pot with the sauce and reheat in preheated oven. Ribs may be prepared up to 3 days in advance and remain in the stock until ready to serve.

Nutrition per Serving
Carbs: 1 g Fiber: 0 g **Net Carbs: 1 g** Protein: 69 g Fat: 169 g Calories: 1853

Beef, Entrées & Main Dishes

Steak au Poivre

Servings: 1

This apart from a simple well seasoned great cut of beef grilled is my favorite recipe for a good quality steak.

There are several fine choices of cuts of steak you could use for this recipe. First of my choice would be a 10 oz. Fillet. My reason for this choice would be that this is an extremely tender cut and prepares very well in this style of preparation. Also the mild flavor always the peppercorns to standout as the main flavoring agent in this dish. Any tender quality cut will work such as center cut strip steaks; center cut rib eye and T-bone or porterhouse.

When choosing a peppercorn for this recipe you will discover that most supermarkets carry a selection of which to choose. I prefer a blend or 3 peppercorn mixture for this recipe. However a simple black peppercorn will work every bit as well.

The secret to this is the sauce you will prepare in the pan.

This recipe is scaled for one steak. Simply multiply the recipe times the number of servings needed.

1 10 oz. Fillet, or any other steak you choose.
3 tablespoons peppercorns, crushed
1 ounce clarified butter
1 teaspoon Worcestershire sauce
2 tablespoons brandy
4 tablespoons brown stock
2 tablespoons green peppercorns, in brine
4 tablespoons heavy cream

Press the cracked pepper into both sides of the steak.

Heat a frying pan or a cast iron frying pan over a high heat, add the butter and when hot, add the steak. Cook for about 4 minutes on each side.

Set the meat aside to rest. Keep it warm in the oven.

Reduce the heat to medium and add the brandy to the frying pan, scrape up all the meat juices, then add the Worcestershire sauce and brown stock. Whisk to combine and cook until the sauce has reduced by a third.

Pour into the sauce any juices that have seeped from the beef.

Add the green peppercorns and cream and cook for an additional 2 minutes. Season to taste with salt.

Put the steak back into the frying pan with the sauce to warm the meat through. Do not reboil.

If you're using a larger or thicker cut, you may need to finish the steak in a 450 degree oven for an additional 5-8 minutes for medium rare.

Nutrition per Serving
Carbs: 3 g Fiber: 0 g **Net Carbs: 3 g** Protein: 2 g Fat: 50 g Calories: 531

Entrées & Main Dishes, Beef

Southwestern Steak with Chipotle Sauce
Servings: 4

Grilled steaks are always a pleasure especially following a Low Carb Lifestyle. Any quality cut of beefsteak is a good choice for grilling. For this example of grilled steak, I have given you some real kick. Adobo spice can be found in most supermarkets in the specialty section or ethnic area. This recipe works just fine using cayenne pepper if you're unable to find this spice.

4 rib eye steaks, 10 oz. center cut boneless
2 teaspoons adobo spice
1 teaspoon ground cumin
2 teaspoons ground ginger
2 teaspoons dried thyme
Salt and pepper, to taste
Sauce (optional)
1 cup brown stock
2 teaspoons chipotle Chile canned in adobo chopped fine
2 tablespoons butter
1 ounce bourbon
Salt and pepper, to taste

In a small mixing bowl, combine all spices except salt and pepper. Blend well and set aside. Season the steaks on each side with salt and pepper to taste and then coat with an equal amount of the blended spices. These spices will form a, crisp coating on the steak when grilled and help to keep the meat juicy. Allow steaks to sit at room temperature for 1-hour. Preheat barbecue grill according to manufacturer's directions. I recommend if using a charcoal grill to use mesquite chip wood for a true Rio Grande flavor. When the grill is ready, cook steak on each side for 2-3 minutes, turning occasionally, until done to your liking. A steak of about 1 inch in thickness will take approximately 3 minutes per side.

FOR SAUCE
Adobo sauce may be purchased in a can and is merely chipotle peppers minced in sauce. This may be found at most grocery stores or Mexican markets. In a sauté pan melt butter over medium-high heat. Add chipotle peppers and deglaze with bourbon.
Add brown stock and cumin. Bring to a rolling boil, cook 2-3 minutes and season lightly with salt and pepper. When steak is done, serve with generous portion of chipotle sauce.

Nutrition per Serving
Carbs: 1 g Fiber: 1 g **Net Carbs: 0 g** Protein: trace g Fat: 6g Calories: 76

Entrées & Main Dishes, Beef

Weekend Barbecued Brisket

Servings: 12

Most backyard cooks shy away from brisket because they fear the tough nature of the meat will come back to ruin a great social affair. In this recipe, the brisket is first braised to tenderness and then finished over a wood fire to guarantee the great freshness and that wonderful outdoor pit flavor. For this example we will use two methods of cooking, both Moist heat and Dry heat (Grilling)

1 whole beef brisket, 7-9 pounds
1 tablespoon kosher salt
1 tablespoon black pepper
2 whole onion, quartered
2 stalks celery
1 head garlic, halved
3 whole bay leaves
1/4 cup old bay Seafood seasoning
Rub
1 tablespoon kosher salt
1 tablespoon chili powder
2 tablespoons sugar twin brown sugar
1 tablespoon black pepper
1 tablespoon ground cumin
1/4 cup Worcestershire sauce

In a large stockpot, combine brisket with 1 tbsp kosher salt, 1 tbsp black pepper, onions, celery, garlic, bay leaves and old bay seasoning. Add cold water to cover brisket by 6-inches. Bring to a rolling boil, reduce to simmer and cook until brisket is fork tender but not falling apart, approximately 1 1/2 - 2 hours depending on the size of the meat. When tender, remove from stock and cool. This may be done one day before grilling. When ready to grill, place coals on one side of the barbecue pit and light according to the manufacturers directions. This will leave the opposite side of the grill cool to place the brisket during smoking. Soak an ample supply of your favorite smoke wood in water and set aside. In a small bowl, combine the remaining salt, Chile powder, brown sugar twin, black pepper and cumin. Blend well to create a seasoning rub. Place the brisket on a large cookie sheet and coat each side in the Worcestershire sauce. Spread the seasoning mixture evenly over each side of the brisket. Using a pair of tongs, place the seasoned brisket directly over the white-hot coals to sear the meat and set the flavor, approximately 3-5 minutes on each side. When the meat has been seared and browned, remove it to the cool side of the pit and place a few handfuls of smoke wood over the hot coals. Close the lid and allow the brisket to smoke off the direct heat until full flavored and heated thoroughly, about 1-hour. Slice and serve with Low Carb barbecue sauce or any other Low Carb salsa.

Nutrition per Serving
Carbs: 2 g Fiber: 1 g **Net Carbs: 1 g** Protein: 4 g Fat: 5 g Calories: 78

Entrées & Main Dishes, Beef

Grilled Veal Chop with Morel Sauce

Servings: 2

Ask your butcher to French these chops for a gourmet look that your guest will marvel at.

4 veal chops, 3/4
OR
2 veal chops, 1 1/4 thick
2 ounces morels, dried
1/4 cup shallots, chopped
1 tablespoon thyme, chopped
1/4 cup white wine
1 cup brown stock
1/2 cup heavy cream
Salt and pepper, to taste

Carefully wash the morels in cold water and allow them to soak for 3 hours. Remove and dry thoroughly. Leave them whole if they are small; cut them up if they are large. In a small sauté pan, melt butter over a medium-high heat. Add shallots and thyme leaves and sauté 2-3 minutes. Add mushrooms and cook another 2-3 minutes.
Deglaze with white wine, and then add brown stock. Reduce to 1/2 volume and season to taste using salt and pepper.
Add cream and continue to cook until sauce is thick enough to coat the back of a spoon. Heat your grill according to manufacturer's directions until coals are white hot. You might wish to add a handful of your favorite smoke wood. Season the chops well with salt and pepper. Grill to your desired doneness. Smaller chops should cook 3-5 minutes on each side for medium-rare, thicker chops should cook 7-9 minutes on each side. Serve with a generous portion of morel sauce.

Nutrition per Serving
Carbs: 8 g Fiber: 1 g **Net Carbs: 7 g** Protein: 73 g Fat: 57 g Calories: 864

Appetizers & Snacks, Beef

Easy Homemade Beef Jerky

Servings: 30

1 1/2 pounds flank steak
1 teaspoon liquid smoke flavoring
1/3 teaspoon garlic powder
1/4 cup soy sauce
1/2 teaspoon black pepper
1 teaspoon onion powder
1 teaspoon Accent® seasoning
1/4 cup Worcestershire sauce

Trim all fat from flank steak. Semi-freeze meat, slice 1/8 inch thick. Combine all ingredients to make marinate.
Marinate overnight in refrigerator. Turn occasionally. Drain well on paper towels, pat dry. Lay on an oven rack.
Do NOT overlap. Place a cookie sheet on lower oven rack to catch drips. Roast at 125 to 140 degrees for 8 to 10 hours. Leave oven door slightly ajar, test for doneness. Store in a brown paper bag or zip lock bag in a dry cool area.

Nutrition per Serving
Carbs: 1 g Fiber: 0 g **Net Carbs: 1 g** Protein: 5 g Fat: 2 g Calories: 43

LAMB

Entrées & Main Dishes, Lamb

Braised Lamb Shanks
Servings: 4

Flavorful and inexpensive dish, your guest will think you took great efforts to create such flavor.
Cooking time will vary depending on the size of the shanks. Always check them as they cook to make certain they do not fall apart during cooking.

8 lamb shanks
1/4 cup olive oil
1 bay leaf
2 celery ribs, chopped
1/2 whole onion, chopped
1 leek, chopped white part only

1 tablespoon rosemary, chopped
1 tablespoon thyme, chopped
1/4 cup red wine
6 cups brown stock
Salt and pepper, to taste

Brown the lamb shanks in enough hot oil to cover the bottom of a large sauté pan. Do not crowd the pan, brown in batches is necessary. Remove shanks and drain well on paper towels.

Place browned lamb shanks in either a deep baking dish or a Dutch oven with a tight fitting lid. Add the bay leaf and the chopped vegetables. Add the brown stock, cover and cook in a 350 degree oven covered for approx 2 hours. Check the lamb after 90 minutes, the meat should be nearly falling of the bone. If not continue to cook till such time.

Once the lamb shanks are tender, remove from pan with tongs, being careful not to let them fall completely apart.

Skim off as much fat as possible from the brown stock.

To serve place 2 shanks per person in either a wide shallow bowl or on a dinner plate. Spoon sauce and vegetables over each. Serve hot with mock potatoes.

Nutrition per Serving
Carbs: 7 g Fiber: 2 g **Net Carbs: 5 g** Protein: 11 g Fat: 21 g Calories: 272

Gregory Pryor C.E.C.

Entrées & Main Dishes, Lamb

Roasted Leg of Lamb (Whole)

Servings: 8

I typically prefer domestic lamb, which often may be a bit larger than most would use for 8 servings. However there are many great uses for left over lamb, such as shepherds pie or simply reheat and serve again.
Have your butcher remove the excess fat from the lamb. Be certain you ask the weight of the lamb so you can determine the proper cooking time.

1 whole leg of lamb, bone in
1/2 cup olive oil
1/4 cup lemon juice
1/2 cup garlic, minced
2 tablespoons rubber sage
2 tablespoons rosemary sprigs, chopped
2 tablespoons thyme, fresh
4 whole bay leaf, whole
8 whole rosemary sprigs
1/2 cup dry red wine
Salt and pepper, to taste

Preheat oven to 350 degrees F. Place the lamb in a large baking pan and rub with olive oil and lemon juice. Using a paring knife, make 8-10 (1-inch) slits on top of the lamb and stuff generously with salt, pepper, 1/4 cup garlic and 2 tablespoons sage. Season the outside of the roast thoroughly with salt, pepper, 2 tablespoons chopped rosemary, 2 tablespoons thyme leaves and remaining garlic. Place the 4 bay leaves in the bottom of the roasting pan and insert 8-10 sprigs of rosemary into each of the seasoned slits. Place lamb in oven and roast 11-13 minutes per pound or until internal temperature reaches 150 degrees F for medium. Remove pan from oven, remove lamb from pan and keep warm. Allow lamb to rest 30 minutes before slicing. Place baking pan on stove top over medium heat. Remove as much fat as possible from the pan, saving the drippings. Deglaze with 1/2 cup red wine, scraping all particles from the bottom of the pan and reduce the liquid by half. Strain sauce through a fine mess strainer and serve alongside the lamb.

Nutrition per Serving
Carbs: 6 g Fiber: 2 g **Net Carbs: 4 g** Protein: 2 g Fat: 15 g Calories: 169

Entrées & Main Dishes, Lamb

Boneless Roasted Leg of Lamb
Servings: 6

This is an item I cannot say enough about. When I was Executive Chef of a prominent Country Club we served this every other week as a carved item on the lunch buffet. We always sold out, and I was partially to blame, I just can't get enough of this marvelous roasted leg of Lamb. At home I serve this with a minted simple brown stock reduction and mock horseradish smashers with green beans.
I prefer domestic Lamb, however the import Lamb is much better these days and milder than it was many years ago.
Be certain to know the weight of the Lamb before you get home, as this will determine the cooking time. Typically domestic boneless Lamb will weight 5-7 pounds while import is usually 3-4 1/2 pounds.

8 slices bacon
1/4 cup olive oil
1 whole boneless leg of lamb
1 bunch fresh rosemary sprigs
Salt and pepper
1 large onion, thinly sliced

Heat a medium skillet over medium-low heat. Place the bacon in the pan and cook until some of the fat is rendered but the bacon has not browned. Drain bacon on paper towels. Preheat oven to 350° F.
Rub the lamb with the olive oil, and season with salt and pepper. Allow lamb to reach room temperature and let stand for 1-hour.
Place lamb in a heavy roasting pan. Arrange bacon over top of lamb in a crisscross pattern. Top with the onion slices. Cook 15 minutes.
Remove lamb from oven, and scatter the rosemary springs over the lamb and around it in the roasting pan.
Return to oven and baste every 20 minutes with the pan drippings. Continue cooking until an instant-read thermometer inserted in the thickest part reads 150° F, about 1-hour and 15 minutes. If the pan juices evaporate, add some stock or water to the roasting pan. Transfer the lamb to a platter. Serve with mint infused reduced brown stock.
To make mint infused brown stock, add 2 cups stock to a saucepot, bring to a simmer and add 6 to 8 sprigs of fresh mint. Reduce stock by 1/3 till slightly thick. Serve hot.

Nutrition per Serving
Carbs: 2 g Fiber: 0 g **Net Carbs: 2 g** Protein: 3 g Fat: 13 g Calories: 136

Entrées & Main Dishes, Lamb

Shepherds Pie
Servings: 6

Here is a classical use for left over lamb. If you don't have left over lamb, most butcher shops will have cubed lamb. You can substitute tender cubed beef for lamb.
I enjoy adding 6-8 large quartered mushrooms to the mixture just before covering with the mock potatoes.

3 cups lamb, cooked and chopped
2 cloves garlic, peeled
1 medium onion, quartered
1 teaspoon rosemary, crumbled
4 ounces butter
2 tablespoons ThickenThin®
3/4 cup brown stock or beef broth
2 cups mock mashed potatoes, or as needed
4 tablespoons clarified butter

Preheat oven to 325°. In a mixing bowl, combine lamb, garlic, onion and rosemary. Put combined ingredients in a food processor and pulse till ingredients are fine chopped. You can alternately chop this with a large kitchen knife. In a skillet with medium heat, melt butter and stir in ThickenThin®. Cook a few minutes until smooth and blended. Slowly add brown stock or beef broth. Stir and cook until thickened, about 5 minutes. Add lamb mixture to the skillet. Stir to blend. Season to taste with salt and pepper. Spoon the skillet's contents into 1 1/2-quart casserole or deep pie dish. Spread mock potatoes on top and cover evenly to the edge of the casserole dish. Drizzle top with clarified butter. Bake at 325° for 45 to 50 minutes, or until meat is bubbling hot and mock potatoes are browned.

Nutrition per Serving
Carbs: 2 g Fiber: 0 g **Net Carbs: 2 g** Protein: 16 g Fat: 35 g Calories: 388

Entrées & Main Dishes, Lamb

Simple Grilled or Roasted Rack of Lamb
Servings: 4

A sophisticated roast that makes a beautiful presentation and is easy to carve. At its best when either grilled or simply oven roasted and served medium rare.
Often I see Frenched racks of lamb packaged in pairs. These are a fine choice as most are in a vacuum packaging and are oven ready.
If the heavy outer layer of fat is intact on the racks use a sharp boning knife and remove the heavy outer layer of fat, or what's known as the cap.
If you shop at a butcher shop the counter man should be happy to French the racks for you.
This is a dish that serving simple sautéed greens adds a full dimension to your meal.

2 whole racks of lamb, frenched
1/4 cup olive oil
2 tablespoons fresh rosemary, chopped
2 tablespoons fresh thyme, chopped
Salt and pepper, to taste

Trim the lamb, if necessary, and rub both sides of the rack with olive oil. Sprinkle with rosemary, thyme, salt and pepper, rubbing them into the meatiest parts of the racks.
Prepare a charcoal or gas grill. Lightly spray the grill rack with vegetable oil cooking spray. The coals should be moderately hot to hot.
Grill the racks, meat side down, for 4 or 5 minutes, or until the temperature of the meatiest part reaches 100 F. Move the racks to the edge of the grill, away from the hottest part of the fire, and cook, covered, for 15 to 20 minutes longer, or until the temperature reaches 140 F for rare meat. Remove the racks from the grill and let them rest for five minutes before cutting between the ribs into individual chops OR preheat your oven to 400 degrees, and place Lamb racks on either a broiler pan or baking sheet fat side up.
Roast 30- 40 minutes till desired doneness. Lamb should always be served no more than medium.

Nutrition per Serving
Carbs: trace g Fiber: 0 g **Net Carbs: trace g** Protein: 52 g Fat: 118 g Calories: 1285

PORK

Entrées & Main Dishes, Pork

Italian Style Pork Stir-Fry

Servings: 4

Stir fry's are simple, filling and always popular, but best of all fast and simple to prepare.

1 medium onion, thinly sliced
1 small red pepper, cut into thin strips
1 teaspoon Italian seasoning
3/4 teaspoon salt
1/3 cup water
1 teaspoon ThickenThin®
1 pound pork tenderloin

1 small eggplant
1 medium summer squash
2 tablespoons olive oil, divided
3/4 teaspoon salt
1/8 teaspoon pepper
1 clove garlic, minced

Partially freeze tenderloin; cut pork diagonally into 1/4-inch thick slices; quarter the slices. Cut squash and eggplant lengthwise in half. Place on flat sides and cut crosswise into 1/4-inch-thick slices. In a skillet, brown half the pork in 1 tablespoon hot olive oil, stirring constantly; remove from pan.
Add the remaining pork; cook, stirring constantly till pork is browned. Sprinkle 3/4 teaspoon salt and the pepper over pork. Place the remaining olive oil, eggplant and minced garlic in skillet and cook over medium-high heat for 3 minutes.
Add squash, onion, red pepper, Italian seasoning, and 3/4 teaspoon salt; cook for 7 minutes, stirring occasionally. Combine water and ThickenThin®; stir into vegetables. Return pork to skillet and cook for 3-4 minutes or till thickened, stirring occasionally.

Nutrition per Serving
Carbs: 14 g Fiber: 5 g **Net Carbs: 9 g** Protein: 26 g Fat: 11 g Calories: 256

Entrées & Main Dishes, Pork

Pork Chops in Low Carb Dill-Sour Cream Sauce

Servings: 6

6 boneless pork chops, 3/4-inch thick
1 1/2 cups sliced fresh mushrooms
1/2 cup thinly sliced green onion
2 teaspoons butter
Salt and pepper
1/2 cup dry white wine OR 1/2 cup chicken stock or 1/4 cup each
1 teaspoon dried dill weed
1 teaspoon Worcestershire sauce
8-ounces sour cream
1/3 cup water
2 tablespoons ThickenThin®

In a large nonstick skillet cook mushrooms and green onions in the butter over medium heat until tender. Remove from skillet; set aside.
Sprinkle chops with salt and pepper. In the same skillet brown chops on each side. Return mushrooms to skillet and add wine, dill, and Worcestershire sauce. Cover tightly; cook over low heat for 5-6 minutes until chops are just done. Remove chops from skillet, keep warm.
In a small bowl combine sour cream, water and ThickenThin®. Stir into skillet; cook over low heat, stirring constantly, until sauce thickens.

Nutrition per Serving
Carbs: 3 g Fiber: 0 g **Net Carbs: 3 g** Protein: 23 g Fat: 16 g Calories: 251

Entrées & Main Dishes, Pork

Pork Chops with Fresh White Mushrooms and Tomato Chutney

Servings: 4

12 ounces fresh white mushrooms
2 tablespoons olive oil, divided
2 large garlic cloves, halved
4 loin pork chops, 3/4-inch thick (about 2 1/2 pounds, bone-in, or 2 pounds, boneless), fat trimmed
1/4 cup dry white wine
1/2 teaspoon salt
1/4 teaspoon red pepper flakes (optional)
1/2 cup plum tomatoes, coarsely chopped
1 large yellow or green bell pepper cut in 1/4-inch strips

Trim mushroom stems; cut in thick slices; set aside. In a large skillet, over medium heat, heat 1 tablespoon of the olive oil until hot. Add garlic; cook and stir until golden, 1 to 2 minutes; remove garlic and discard. In the same skillet, cook pork chops until lightly browned, turning once, 6 to 8 minutes; remove and set aside. Raise heat to medium high; add wine, salt and red pepper flakes (if using). Cook, stirring to loosen particles, until wine is reduced by half, 2 to 3 minutes. Add tomatoes and return chops to skillet. Reduce heat to low, cover and simmer, basting occasionally, until chops are tender, about 15 minutes. Meanwhile, in a medium-size skillet, over medium heat, heat remaining 1 tablespoon olive oil until hot. Add reserved mushrooms and the bell pepper; cook and stir until vegetables are softened, about 5 minutes. Add mushroom mixture to skillet with pork chops. Cover and simmer mixture just until hot, about 3 minutes, adding 1 to 2 tablespoons water if needed.

Nutrition per Serving
Carbs: 7 g Fiber: 2 g **Net Carbs: 5 g** Protein: 21 g Fat: 12 g Calories: 234

Gregory Pryor C.E.C.

Entrées & Main Dishes, Pork

Pork Piccata
Servings: 4

1 1/2 pounds boneless pork tenderloin
1 1/2 teaspoons lemon pepper
2 tablespoons clarified butter
1/4 cup lemon juice
1/4 cup white wine
4 thin lemon slices (4 to 6 slices)
1/4 cup capers

Slice Pork tenderloin into 4 equal pieces. Pound cutlets thin (about 1/8" thick) evenly. Season with lemon pepper.
Melt butter in large skillet over medium-high heat. Quickly sauté cutlets, turning once, until golden-brown, about 5-6 minutes. Add wine and lemon juice to skillet; shake pan gently and cook 2-3 minutes, until sauce is slightly reduced. Serve cutlets garnished with lemon slices and capers.

Nutrition per Serving
Carbs: 3g Fiber: 0 g **Net Carbs: 3g** Protein: 22 Fat: 12 Calories: 214

Entrées & Main Dishes, Pork

Pork Scaloppini with Creamy Caper Sauce
Servings: 6

Most every butcher shop with have pork scaloppini. If not ask the butcher to cut and pound them for you. This same procedure is repeated for many other dishes such as, chicken, veal and turkey. So feel free to substitute any other scaloppini.

2 1/2 pounds pork tenderloins (about 2 whole)
2 tablespoons clarified butter
1/4 teaspoon salt
2/3 cup dry white wine
2/3 cup light cream
1 clove garlic, minced (optional)
Or replace garlic with minced shallot
1/8 teaspoon white pepper
2 tablespoons capers, drained

Cut each tenderloin crosswise into six 1-inch thick slices. With a meat mallet or cleaver, pound each slice to 1/2-inch thickness.
In a large skillet cook pork medallions in hot butter over medium heat about 3-4 minutes on each side. Remove pork to a warm platter; season with salt. Keep warm.
For the sauce, add wine to skillet drippings. Bring to boiling, scraping up any browned bits in skillet. Add cream, garlic and pepper. Cook and stir 3 minutes or until thickened. Remove from heat, stir in capers. To serve, pour sauce over pork.

Nutrition per Serving
Carbs: 1 g Fiber: 0 g **Net Carbs: 1 g** Protein: 25 g Fat: 9 g Calories: 207

Gregory Pryor C.E.C.

Entrées & Main Dishes, Pork

Country Ribs and Sauerkraut
Servings: 4

This simple recipe is better when prepared the day before, and reheated the next day.
I prepare this on the weekend and keep it in the fridge to use for dinner any week day. After the recipe is completely cooled I store the entire recipe in a gallon zip lock bag. When ready to use just place in a baking dish and heat thru till steaming hot.
When shopping for sauerkraut make certain to read the label closely. The fresh, not canned is generally the lowest in Carbs. However I have seen several brands in large jars that also are low in Carbs. Choose wisely.

3 pounds country style ribs
1 pound sauerkraut, see notes
1 large onion, chopped
1 tablespoon caraway seeds
Salt and pepper, to taste

Season country style ribs well with salt and pepper. In a large skillet, brown the ribs. I like these well browned. It makes a big difference in the final dish if these are very brown. Remove from skillet and allow to drain. Place the kraut in a baking dish large enough to hold the kraut and ribs. Lay the browned ribs evenly over the kraut. Sprinkle with the caraway seeds. Cover with foil and bake at 350 for approx. 45-60 minutes. Remove and serve or let cool and save for another time.

Nutrition per Serving
Carbs: 8 g Fiber: 4 g **Net Carbs: 4 g** Protein: 2 g Fat: 3 g Calories: 138

Entrées & Main Dishes, Pork

Skillet Pork Chops Dijon Style
Servings: 4

Thick pork chops with creamy Dijon sauce. This same recipe works well with skin on chicken breast. Simply season each breast and cook in the same way as described here. Skins on breast are the better choice for flavor and presentation. Be certain to start the breast skin side down and cook till skin is a golden-brown and crisp. Then turn breast and continue with recipe.

4 pork loin chops, 3/4 - to 1-inch thick
1 tablespoon olive oil
Salt and white pepper, to taste
1 tablespoon shallot, finely minced
1/8 teaspoon sage
1 cup chicken stock or broth
FOR SAUCE
2 tablespoons ThickenThin®
1/2 cup half-and-half
1 1/2 tablespoons Dijon mustard, or to taste
GARNISH
1/2 cup parsley, finely chopped

Slash fat surrounding chops to prevent curling. Season with salt and pepper. Heat oil in heavy skillet on medium-high heat. Add chops to pan, cooking approximately 5 minutes per side. Add chicken stock or broth, shallots, and sage; bring to boil.
Cover; simmer for 20-30 minutes, depending on the thickness of the chops.
FOR SAUCE:
Remove chops from pan, keep warm. Remove pan from heat.
Wisk in ThickenThin® and the half-and-half together, removing all lumps. Add the mixture to the pan, stirring constantly until blended with the broth.
Return to medium-high heat. Add the mustard and continue to stir until thickened and bubbly, about 1-minute.
Place chops on plate and spoon a portion of the sauce over them, reserving the remaining sauce to pass. Sprinkle with chopped parsley.
Serving Ideas: Serve with any green vegetable and use the extra sauce for the vegetables.

Nutrition per Serving
Carbs: 3 g Fiber: 0 g **Net Carbs: 3 g** Protein: 21 g Fat: 16g Calories: 241

Entrées & Main Dishes, Pork

Southwestern Pork Loin

Servings: 6

4 pounds boneless pork loin roast, trimmed
1 tablespoon olive oil
2 cups tomatoes (about 2 medium), chopped and seeded
1 medium onion, chopped
1/2 cup chopped fresh cilantro
1 Tomatillo (about 1/3 cup), peeled, chopped (optional)
4 cloves garlic, minced
1 jalapeño pepper, chopped, seeded (optional)
1 4-ounce can chopped green chilies, drained
1/2 teaspoon dried oregano leaves
1/2 teaspoon ground cumin
1/2 teaspoon ground red pepper
1/2 teaspoon ground coriander

Heat oil in a large skillet over medium heat. Add tomatoes, onion, cilantro, Tomatillo, garlic, jalapeño pepper and chilies; cook about 2 minutes or until onion is tender, stirring frequently. Add oregano, cumin, red pepper and coriander; mix well. Refrigerate mixture until thoroughly chilled.

Heat oven to 325ºF. Spray shallow baking pan with nonstick cooking spray. Using sharp knife, cut 8-10 slits about 1 inch long and 1 inch deep in top and sides of pork roast. Press heaping teaspoonful of cold vegetable mixture into each slit; spread remaining mixture over top and sides of roast. Place in prepared pan. Roast for about 1 ½ hours, or until meat thermometer registers 155ºF. Let stand 10 minutes before slicing.

Nutrition per Serving
Carbs: 7 g Fiber: 2 g **Net Carbs: 5 g** Protein: 61 g Fat: 24 g Calories: 458

Entrées & Main Dishes, Pork

Stuffed Pork Loin
Servings: 6

Pork loin for my money is one of the best products likely found in either the local butcher shop or supermarket.
This is just one of several examples of the use of pork loin we will use throughout the book. Served with a little mushroom sauce and a side. Practice your plate presentation and impress your family or guest. Slice 3 or 4, 1-1/2 to 2 inch think slices per serving. Spoon 2 tablespoons of mushroom sauce just off center of the plate then lay the pork slices over the sauce in a small spiral shingled layer following the curve of the dinner plate. Serve with a generous scoop of mock mashed potatoes in the center of the dinner plate, and a serving of garlicky green beans opposite the pork. Shake a little paprika over entire dish and serve. Your family and guest will be delighted at your culinary skill.

2 pounds single pork loin roast
1/2 cup chopped onion
2 cloves garlic, minced
OR
1 teaspoon bottled minced garlic
1 tablespoon olive oil
1/2 10-ounce package frozen chopped spinach, thawed, well drained
6 slices bacon, cooked well done, drained and crumbled
3 tablespoons grated Parmesan cheese
1 tablespoon Dijon-style mustard
1/4 cup basil, chopped
1/4 teaspoon pepper

Butterfly pork loin by cutting roast horizontally to within 1/4-inch of the other side. Do not cut all the way through. Open out and pound to 8 × 8-inch rectangle.
Meanwhile, cook onion and garlic in hot oil until tender; remove from heat. Press well-drained spinach between several sheets of paper towels to remove moisture. Add to onion mixture along with crumbled bacon, Parmesan cheese, mustard, basil and pepper. Mix well. Spread spinach mixture on pork rectangle. Roll up into a spiral. Tie with kitchen string to secure.
Place pork in shallow pan and roast in a 350 degree F. oven for 45-50 minutes, until internal temperature (Measured with a meat thermometer) reads 155ºF. Remove from oven, let rest 5 minutes. Slice to serve, removing string.

Nutrition per Serving
Carbs: 4 g Fiber: 2 g **Net Carbs: 2 g** Protein: 34 g Fat: 17 g Calories: 289

Entrées & Main Dishes, Pork

Easy Roast Suckling Pig
Servings: 14

Baking Time: 6 hours
Planning a backyard cook out, or do you just want to dazzle your guest at a casual diner party. No matter what the occasion, this is always a crowd pleaser. Do not be intimidated by this at all, it is no more work than cooking a turkey. Many major supermarkets will order the pig for you or ask your butcher shop operator to do so.
Should you have any leftovers, let cool and remove and "pull" the pork to make pulled pork for another dish. Mix pulled pork with Low Carb BBQ sauce and serve with basic Cole slaw for a classical southern style dish.

1 16-pound whole pig cleaned and ready to cook
1 teaspoon salt
6 cloves garlic
1 tablespoon salt
1/2 loaf unsliced bread
1 apple

The pig should weigh about 16 pounds. Wash it thoroughly and drain. Salt it inside and outside generously. Cut slits under the shoulders and on the thighs. Put 1 teaspoon salt and a cut piece of garlic in each slit. Put 6 cloves of garlic and 1 tablespoon salt in a clean cloth. Pound this slightly with a hammer. Rub cloth over pig inside and outside. Put 1/2 loaf of un-sliced bread inside pig. In your largest roasting pan, place 2 short pieces of clean board.
(So the roast won't stick to bottom of pan). Cover top of pig with foil or heavy parchment paper. Place shiny apple in the mouth. Bake at 350 for 5 to 6 hrs, basting with oil or beer once or twice. It is done when no pink juice runs when pierced with fork. Remove bread and dispose of it. Serve hot or cold. If apple becomes soft after baking, replace with a fresh one.

Nutrition per Serving
Carbs: 2 g Fiber: 0 g **Net Carbs: 2 g** Protein: 74 g Fat: 81 g Calories: 1065

POULTRY

Entrées & Main Dishes, Poultry

Chicken Skillet Dinner

Servings: 4

1/2 cup chicken stock
1 tablespoon cornstarch
1 tablespoon soy sauce
1/2 teaspoon ground ginger
3 tablespoons vegetable oil, divided
1 pound boned and skinned chicken breasts, cut into thin slices
2 teaspoons minced garlic
6 ounces radishes, sliced (about 1 1/2 cups)
1/4 cup sliced green onions (scallions)

In a small bowl, combine chicken stock, cornstarch, soy sauce and ginger until smooth; set aside. In a large skillet, heat 2 tablespoons of the oil over high heat until hot. Add chicken and garlic; cook, stirring constantly, just until chicken is cooked through, about 3 minutes. Remove from skillet; set aside. Add remaining 1 tablespoon oil; heat until hot. Stir in radishes and green onions; cook and stir for 1-minute; remove from heat. Return chicken to skillet.

Stir broth mixture; pour into skillet and bring to a boil. Boil and stir until sauce is clear and slightly thickened, about 1-minute. Serve over sautéed fresh bean sprouts, if desired.

Nutrition per Serving
Carbs: 4 g Fiber: 1 g **Net Carbs: 3 g** Protein: 27 g Fat: 12 g Calories: 238

Gregory Pryor C.E.C.

Entrées & Main Dishes, Poultry

Coq Au Vin
Servings: 4

This classical chicken recipe was always made with a large baking hen or rooster. These days we use a large baking hen. I have done this dish using a Capon; however I prefer the baking hen. The increased cooking time ensures much better flavor because of the marriage of meat, vegetables and wine. Should you choose to use a smaller frying chicken, be careful of the cooking time. The bird will fall apart, and the full flavor does not develop. Classically in this dish we would use pearl onions and sweet peas, as you will see for our Low Carb version I have adjusted a few of the classical items to lower the Carb count.

When chicken quarters are on sale, normally these quarters are from large stewing hens. Look for those when offered. I know in our area often I see 10 pound bags of quarters for .49 cents a pound. These work great for this dish. Simply cut each at the joint. You can freeze what you have left for either grilling or baking at another time.

1 large whole chicken (stewing) cut into 8 pieces
1/2 cup clarified butter
3/4 cup onion, chopped
3/4 cup celery, chopped
1/4 cup garlic, diced
3/4 cup dry red wine
2 cups chicken stock
20 small button mushrooms
1 tablespoon thyme, chopped
1 tablespoon rosemary, chopped
1 whole bay leaf
Salt and pepper, to taste

Cut hen into 8 serving pieces. In a heavy-bottomed Dutch oven, heat clarified butter over medium-high heat. Season chicken with salt and pepper. Brown on both sides, remove and set aside. Add celery, garlic and onions. Sauté 3 to 5 minutes or until vegetables are wilted.
Return chicken to pot and add red wine and chicken stock. Bring to a rolling boil and reduce to simmer. Add mushrooms, thyme, oregano and bay leaf, adjust seasonings if necessary. Cover and braise for 1-hour and check for tenderness. You may need to skim any fats that rise to the surface during the cooking.

Nutrition per Serving
Carbs: 14 g Fiber: 6 g **Net Carbs: 8 g** Protein: 38 g Fat: 36 g Calories: 595

Entrées & Main Dishes, Poultry

Fried Chicken

Servings: 4

For best results, heat the butter temperature between 350 degrees F and 360 degrees F. Also, 2 cups buttermilk may be substituted for the saltwater solution used to soak the chicken pieces.

We will be using our own fresh almond flour for this recipe, here are a few tips. For best results use sliced blanched almonds. In a food processor pulse grind the almonds. For this example the flour need not be perfectly fine.

A little course texture improves the "crunch" of the chicken. When browning the chicken in the clarified butter or oil, do not try to completely cook the chicken and be certain not to over brown the chicken as we will finish cooking the chicken in the oven.

Another tip for fried chicken; you can create a crispy flavorful fried chicken without any coating at all. I fry fresh dry chicken skin-on in clarified butter. Simply season chicken well, sprinkle with a little paprika and fry over medium high heat, turning chicken often till crispy and brown and cooked through.

3 quarts water
3 tablespoons kosher salt
1 whole chicken, 3 to 3 1/2 pounds cut into 8 pieces
1 tablespoon salt
1 tablespoon black pepper
1 cup almond slivers, ground (see notes)
1 cup clarified butter

Combine 3 quarts water and 1 tablespoon salt in a large bowl or buttermilk; add chicken pieces. Cover and refrigerate 8 hours or overnight. Drain chicken; if having used the salted water rinse with cold water and pat dry, if using the buttermilk (my choice) then let chicken drain. Combine 1 teaspoon salt and 1 teaspoon pepper; sprinkle half of mixture over all sides of chicken. Combine remaining mixture and almond flour in a gallon-size, heavy-duty, zip-lock plastic bag. Place 2 pieces of chicken in bag; seal. Shake to coat completely. Remove chicken, and repeat procedure with remaining pieces. Add clarified butter to a 12-inch cast-iron skillet or large heavy bottom sauté pan over medium heat. Add chicken, a few pieces at a time, skin side down. Brown chicken evenly on all side, do not overcook. Once all chicken pieces are a golden-brown place in a preheated 350 degree oven for approx 20 - 30 minutes to finish.

Nutrition per Serving
Carbs: 5 g Fiber: 2 g **Net Carbs: 3 g** Protein: 72 g Fat: 128 g Calories: 1469

Gregory Pryor C.E.C.

Entrées & Main Dishes, Poultry

Chicken Piccata
Servings: 4

4 boneless skinless breasts chicken
1/2 cup clarified butter
1 tbsp minced garlic
1/2 cup dry white wine
1 cup chicken broth or chicken stock
3 tablespoon fresh lemon juice
2 tablespoon capers, drained
4 lemon slices, thinly cut
4 tablespoon unsalted butter
1/4 cup chopped parsley
Salt and pepper to taste

Slice each chicken breast in half. Place chicken halves between sheets of plastic wrap and pound to an even thickness. Season chicken to taste with salt and pepper. In a large sauté pan, heat clarified butter over medium-high heat. Sauté cutlets a few at a time, 2-3 minutes on each side. Remove cutlets from pan and pour off all but 2 tablespoons of butter. Add garlic and sauté one minute. Deglaze with white wine. Bring to a rolling boil and reduce to half volume. Add chicken stock, lemon juice, capers and lemon slices. Return chicken to the pan and simmer in stock for 1-2 minutes or until heated thoroughly. Add the butter and parsley, swirling the pan constantly until butter sauce is achieved. Remove from heat and serve.

Nutrition per Serving
Carbs: 3 g Fiber: 0 g **Net Carbs: 3 g** Protein: 22 g Fat: 12 g Calories: 214

Entrées & Main Dishes, Poultry

Spicy Buffalo Chicken Wings

Servings: 2

*This is the best recipe you will ever need for buffalo wings. I make these 2 - 3 times a week. I can't tell you how many of these I have eaten while writing this book. The 3 key points to this for great wings. 1. I always use fresh medium to large wings. If the wings are too small the cooking time will dry them out. Although I have used the IQF frozen wings and drumettes the quality just isn't as good. These are not bad mind you but here fresh is best. 2. You must use good oil for frying and a good source of heat. If the oil drops to far in temperature the wings will be oily. Start with the oil at 365 and keep the oil on high heat, as the wings cook the temperature will return to 350 to 360 degrees. 3. The sauce. There are many wing sauces on the market, be cautious as many of the bottled wing sauces are high in Carbs. I always make my own. I prefer a bottled sauce called Ricky's hot sauce. Choose a bottled sauce that you like, making certain it is a zero or no more than 1g Carb per serving. Using the sauce of your choice in a saucepan add 2 cups of the sauce. Bring to a simmer and add 1/2 pound of unsalted butter. Allow this to melt and blend slowly. Once blended you can flavor this further if you like. Add 6 cloves of minced garlic for a garlic sauce. Should you like a sweet sauce add 4 tablespoons of Splenda®. If a simple wing sauce is your choice once the butter is blended simply use as is. This keeps nicely in the fridge. Last tip; always use the sauce at room temperature.
Serve with crisp celery and blue cheese dip.*

24 chicken wings, separated at the joint tips discarded or save for stock
4 cups oil, for frying

In a deep fryer such as a fry daddy or a large saucepot, add clean oil and heat to 365 degrees.
Carefully drop the wings into the hot oil and cook till golden-brown and crisp, approx. 12 - 15 minutes.
Drain and in a large metal or ceramic bowl add wings and enough wing sauce to coat. Toss wings several times to coat wings evenly.
Serve piping hot.
If you're using a fry daddy with a storage lid, you can use this oil several times till the oil becomes dark.
You may also want to strain the oil and store in a covered jar in the fridge for up to one month.

Nutrition per Serving
Carbs: 0 g Fiber: 0 g **Net Carbs: 0 g** Protein: 216 g Fat: 188g Calories: 1320

Gregory Pryor C.E.C.

Entrées & Main Dishes, Poultry

Chicken Breasts Diane
Servings: 4

This same preparation can be used with minute steaks to create a simple Steak Diane. For an even larger portion of Steak Diane I suggest using either a boneless 10 oz. Center cut strip or a 10 oz. Rib eye. Sauté the same as the chicken till desired doneness.

4 whole chicken breast halves without skin
1/2 teaspoon Salt
1/2 teaspoon Pepper
2 tablespoons olive oil
2 tablespoons clarified butter
3 tablespoons chives, chopped
1/2 whole lime, juice only (do not substitute)
3 tablespoons parsley, chopped
2 teaspoons Dijon-style mustard
1/4 cup chicken stock

Place the chicken breast halves between sheets of waxed paper.
Pound slightly with a mallet. Sprinkle with salt and pepper.
Heat half the butter and half the olive oil in a large skillet.
Cook the chicken breasts over high heat for 4 minutes on each side.
Transfer to a warm serving platter.
Add the chives, lime juice, brandy, parsley and mustard to the pan.
Cook, whisking constantly, for 15 seconds. Whisk in the stock.
Stir until the sauce is smooth. Whisk in the remaining butter and olive oil.
Pour the sauce over the chicken. Serve at once.

Nutrition per Serving
Carbs: 2 g Fiber: 0 g **Net Carbs: 2 g** Protein: 28 Fat: 110 g Calories: 1095

Entrées & Main Dishes, Poultry

Sautéed Chicken Breast with Green Olives and Cilantro

Servings: 4

This dish may appear a little busy from first glance, however it really is very simple to complete. The flavors and presentation make this all worth the little effort to prepare. I serve this with sautéed Swiss chard for a complete meal

2 whole chicken breasts, skin on, split into 2 halves
3 tablespoons olive oil
1/4 cup onion, minced
2 teaspoons gingerroot, minced
1 pinch saffron threads, optional
2 cups chicken stock
2 tablespoons peanut oil
2 tablespoons green olives, minced
1 tablespoon cilantro leaves, whole, chopped
Salt and pepper, to taste

Preheat the oven to 500°F. Place 2 tablespoons olive oil in a small saucepan over medium heat. Add the onion, ginger and saffron or turmeric and a pinch of salt and cook, stirring occasionally, for about 5 minutes. Add the stock and increase the heat to high; cook, stirring occasionally, while you prepare the chicken. When the liquid has reduced by about three-quarters and becomes syrupy, turn off the heat.

Heat the peanut or other oil in a large, preferably nonstick, ovenproof skillet over medium-high heat for a minute or two. Season the chicken on both sides with salt and pepper. Place the chicken in the skillet, skin side down, and cook undisturbed until lightly browned, 5 to 8 minutes.

Turn over and cook on the other side for about 2 minutes. Turn the chicken skin side down again, and place the skillet in the oven. Check it after 15 minutes, and remove when chicken juices run clear.

When the chicken is just about done, finish the sauce. Stir in the remaining 1 teaspoon of olive oil, the olives and some salt (not too much as the olives are salty) and pepper. Cook for about 2 minutes over medium-high heat stirring once or twice. Turn off the heat and add the lemon juice and cilantro.

To serve, arrange the chicken on 4 plates. Spoon the sauce around it, not over it, so the chicken stays crunchy.

Nutrition per Serving
Carbs: 2 g Fiber: 0 g **Net Carbs: 2 g** Protein: 31 g Fat: 31 g Calories: 419

Gregory Pryor C.E.C.

Entrées & Main Dishes, Poultry

Spicy Blackened Chicken Breasts
Servings: 4

When we blacken any item rather it is chicken or fish nothing works better than a heavy cast iron skillet. If you do not have one of these a heavy bottom fry pan will work.

2 tablespoons paprika
3/4 tablespoon onion powder
3/4 tablespoon garlic powder
3/4 tablespoon cayenne
1/2 tablespoon white pepper
1/2 tablespoon black pepper
1/2 tablespoon thyme, finely chopped
1/2 tablespoon oregano, finely chopped
1/2 tablespoon Salt
4 whole chicken breast halves
4 tablespoons clarified butter

Melt the butter.
The chicken breasts must be skinless and boneless.
Dip the chicken breasts on both sides in the melted butter.
Place on waxed paper.
Combine the spice mix ingredients and sprinkle over both sides of the chicken breasts. Pat the mixture firmly into the meat. Place a large cast iron skillet over medium high heat for 8 minutes. Add the chicken breasts and cook until "*blackened*". Turn the chicken over and cook until it is cooked through (about 10 minutes in all). Serve at once.

Nutrition per Serving
Carbs: 6 g Fiber: 2 g **Net Carbs: 4 g** Protein: 32 g Fat: 27 g Calories: 392

Entrées & Main Dishes, Poultry

Supreme Chicken Breast Amandine
Servings: 4

4 whole chicken breast halves without skin, boneless
8 tablespoons clarified butter
2 tablespoons lemon juice
1/2 cup sliced almonds
1 teaspoon garlic, minced
1 tablespoon onion, minced
1/4 cup dry white wine
Salt and pepper, to taste

Heat half the butter in a heavy skillet.
Season the chicken on both sides and slowly brown the chicken breasts on both sides. Add the lemon juice.
Season with salt and pepper to taste. Cover the pan. Sauté gently until the chicken is tender (10-15 minutes).
Remove the chicken from the skillet.
Add half the remaining butter to the pan. Add the almonds.
Brown them over low heat. Add the onion and garlic.
Cook for 1-minute. Add the wine and the remaining butter.
Return the chicken to the skillet and reheat. Remove from the heat.
Spoon the almonds and sauce over. Sprinkle chopped parsley over.
Serve hot.

Nutrition per Serving
Carbs: 5 g Fiber: 1 g **Net Carbs: 4 g** Protein: 31 g Fat: 36 g Calories: 474

Entrées & Main Dishes, Poultry

Lemon Baked Chicken Breasts

Servings: 4

If whole chicken breasts are difficult to find in a supermarket you can use skin on bone in halves. Ask the butcher if he has whole breast, as these cook better in the oven and have more flavor.

1 tablespoon clarified butter
1 tablespoon olive oil
2 whole chicken breast, about 1 1/4 pounds each
1 cup dry white wine
1/2 teaspoon dried thyme
2 tablespoons lemon juice, fresh

In a large heavy skillet, heat butter and oil over moderately high heat until the foam begins to subside, add the chicken, patted dry, skin side down, and sauté, turning it, until it is golden. Transfer the chicken to a baking dish and pour off the excess fat in the skillet. Add the wine and the thyme to the skillet bring to a boil, scraping up the brown bits, and pour the pan juices over the chicken. Season chicken with salt and pepper, sprinkle it with lemon juice, and bake it in the lower third of a preheated 400 degree oven for 30 minutes, or until it is tender. Remove and split breast into 2 pieces. Serve each half as one portion. Strain any pan juices from the chicken and spoon over each breast.

Nutrition per Serving
Carbs: 1 g Fiber: 0 g **Net Carbs: 1 g** Protein: 30 g Fat: 20 g Calories: 350

Main Dishes, Poultry

Chicken Parmesan Cutlets

Servings: 4

This dish can be prepared using Turkey or Veal.

1/4 cup grated Parmesan cheese
1/8 teaspoon Italian seasoning
1/4 teaspoon seasoned salt
1/4 teaspoon ground black pepper
8 whole chicken breast, no skin, no bone, cutlets cut 1/2-inch thick

Combine cheese, Italian seasoning, salt and pepper in small dish. Place cheese mixture on plate and coat each cutlet. Spray large nonstick skillet with nonstick cooking spray and heat over medium-high heat. Add several cutlets and cook until no longer pink, about 2 minutes per side. Keep cooked cutlets warm. Wipe out skillet, spray again and continue cooking remaining cutlets. Spoon Low Carb fresh tomato sauce over each cutlet. Serve with Caesar salad and your vegetable of choice.

Nutrition per Serving
Carbs: trace g Fiber: 0 g **Net Carbs: trace g** Protein: 107 g Fat: 14 g Calories: 580

Gregory Pryor C.E.C.

Main Dishes, Poultry

Tomato Chicken Grill
Servings: 4

Remember those chicken quarters I talked about before, here is a recipe that works great with those.
Chicken quarters are a true bargain in 10 pound bags at most supermarkets.

4 broiler-fryer chicken quarters
1/4 cup fresh lime juice
1 1/2 teaspoons chopped chives
1 teaspoon freshly grated ginger
2 cloves garlic, minced
2 tablespoons olive oil
1 teaspoon chili powder
1 cup low carb salsa of your choice, see recipes

In small saucepan, mix lime juice, chives, ginger and garlic. Add olive oil and chili powder and heat to boiling over medium heat. Stir in salsa. Place chicken in single layer in large, shallow bowl. Pour sauce over chicken and turn to coat well. Cover and refrigerate at least 2 hours. When ready to cook, place chicken on prepared grill, skin side up, about 8 inches from heat. Grill, turning every 10 minutes, about 1-hour or until fork can be inserted in chicken with ease. Heat marinade to boiling and boil about 3 minutes; pour over chicken.

Nutrition per Serving
Carbs: 2 g Fiber: 0 g **Net Carbs: 2 g** Protein: 20 g Fat: 23 g Calories: 303

Main Dishes, Poultry

Herb Roasted Mushrooms, Chicken and Vegetable Sheppard's Pie

Servings: 4

1/4 cup olive oil
2 teaspoons dried rosemary, crushed
1 1/3 teaspoons salt
1/3 teaspoon ground black pepper
1 pound boneless, skinless chicken breasts cut into 2-1/2 inch pieces
1 pound fresh white mushrooms, halved (about 6 cups)
1 medium onion cut in wedges (about 3 cups)
1 large red bell pepper cut in 2-inch pieces (about 2 cups)
4 large garlic cloves, peeled
2 cups mock mashed potatoes

Preheat oven to 425ºF. In a large bowl combine oil, rosemary, salt and pepper until well blended. Add chicken, mushrooms, onions, red bell pepper and garlic; toss until well coated. Divide mixture into two baking or deep dish pie pans. Roast until chicken and vegetables are tender, about 30 minutes, stirring occasionally and rotating pans on shelves once during roasting. Remove and cover with mock mash potatoes either plain or flavored of your choice. Sprinkle with a little clarified butter and paprika. Place under broiler to brown top and serve hot.

Nutrition per Serving
Carbs: 11 g Fiber: 3 g **Net Carbs: 8 g** Protein: 28 g Fat: 16 g Calories: 293

SEAFOOD

Lobster Cooking Tips

Boiling:

When boiling lobsters, use a kettle large enough to hold 1 or 2 lobsters at a time allowing 3-quarts of water per lobster. You may wish to add 1 tbsp of salt per quart. When water comes to a rolling boil, submerge live lobsters one at a time. Return water to a boil. Lower heat to simmer and boil 8 to 10 minutes for 1 to 1 1/4 pound lobsters, or 12 to 14 minutes for 1 ½ pound lobsters. The tails should begin to float toward the surface once the lobsters are cooked.

Steaming:

If you wish to steam a lobster it is best done in a large stainless steel pasta pot using the steaming insert. Place approximately 2 inches of water in the bottom of the stockpot and bring to a rolling boil. Place 2 or more lobsters in the pot cover and steam 8 to 10 minutes for a 1 to 1 1/4-pound lobster and 12 to 14 minutes for a 1 ½ pound lobster.

Grilling or Broiling:

If you prefer to grill or broil your lobster, I suggest submerging the lobster for 2 minutes into a pot of boiling water. Remove and allow the lobster to cool slightly. Turn the lobster over on its back and, using a sharp chef's knife, split it open from head to tail. Brush the

Gregory Pryor C.E.C.

tail meat lightly with oil or butter and season with salt and pepper. If grilling over either charcoal or a gas grill, lightly oil the grill surface with either vegetable oil or spray with Pam. Place the lobster cut side down on the grill and cook for about 8-10 minutes. Turn over and move to a cooler side of the grill for 5 minutes. Serve with drawn butter. If broiling, place the lobster on a large cookie sheet, meat side down and cook 5 minutes. Turn over onto the shell and cook 5 additional minutes, or until meat is firm and white. As with any seafood, **do not overcook**.

Entrées & Main Dishes, Fish & Seafood

Crab Stuffed Baked Lobster

Servings: 2

For this simple version of baked stuffed lobster be certain to follow the guidelines listed for preparing the lobster for this recipe.

2 whole lobsters, live
Crab stuffing
1/2 cup drawn butter

Crab Stuffing
Shrimp could be substituted for crab.

1 cup cooked flaked crabmeat canned and picked clean is fine.
8 ounces cream cheese, softened
1/4 cup mayonnaise
1 teaspoon lemon juice
2 Dashes Worcestershire sauce
1/4 teaspoon basil
1/4 teaspoon garlic powder
2 green onions, minced
1/8 teaspoon lemon pepper

Combine all stuffing ingredients in a bowl and mix well.

Split a live lobster: Spread flat. Using a teaspoon, remove the tomalley (greenstuff) and coral (pink stuff, roe) and reserve. Remove stomach (under the head) and devein. Leave claws intact. To the crab stuffing add the tomalley and coral, and toss to mix well. Fill the cavity of each lobster with the stuffing.
Place in a foil lined baking pan, alternating head and tail to fit better. Bring the edge of foil up over the tail of each lobster. Press to secure end of tail to pan so the tails do not curl up as they bake. Bake at 325 degrees for 50 minutes, more or less depending on size. Serve straight from the oven.

Nutrition per Serving
Carbs: 3 g Fiber: 0 g **Net Carbs: 3 g** Protein: 3 g Fat: 9 g Calories: 435

Gregory Pryor C.E.C.

Entrées & Main Dishes, Fish & Seafood

Lobster Thermidor

Servings: 2

2 whole lobsters, live
1/4 pound mushrooms, sliced
2 tablespoons clarified butter
2 ounces sherry, optional
1 cup heavy cream
1/4 cup cheddar cheese, grated
3 whole egg yolks, beaten
Paprika
Parmesan cheese
Salt and pepper, to taste

Split and broil lobsters and remove meat. Using a teaspoon, remove the tomalley (greenstuff) and coral (pink stuff, roe) and reserve Empty and clean shells. Reserve shells. Sauté lobster meat and sliced mushrooms in butter for 5 minutes add the tomalley and roe. Add salt and pepper to taste. Add sherry and braise for 2 minutes. Slowly stir in cream bring to a simmer. Add cheese and stir until it melts. Sprinkle with paprika. Remove from heat and blend in egg yolks. Fill lobster shells with the lobster mixture. Sprinkle with Parmesan cheese and a dash of paprika. Place under broiler till brown and bubbly.

Nutrition per Serving
Carbs: 9 g Fiber: 1 g **Net Carbs: 8 g** Protein: 40 g Fat: 71 g Calories: 857

Entrées & Main Dishes, Fish/ Seafood

Poached White Fish with Lemon Butter Sauce

Servings: 6

Any firm white fish may be used. Although water can be used to poach the fish, I prefer to use fish stock. If you don't have fish stock use half water and half white wine.

The most important key to this dish is understanding "simmer". When we poach any item, fish, chicken, even beef, the degree of simmer is critical to recognize. As in this case, the proper simmer is when the liquid just barely bubbles. Any faster simmer or boil will result in a dry and often tough product, especially chicken and beef items. Try adding a tablespoon of capers to the lemon sauce.

1 1/2 pounds firm white fish, cod, grouper, Sea bass, etc, thawed if necessary
1 quart water
1/4 cup lemon juice
1 small onion, sliced
1 bay leaf
4 peppercorns
4 whole cloves
1 teaspoon salt
LEMON BUTTER SAUCE
1/4 cup butter
2 tablespoons lemon juice
Minced parsley

Cut fish into serving-size pieces. Combine water, lemon juice, onion and seasonings. Bring to boil; simmer 20 minutes. Add fish pieces. (If necessary, add boiling water to cover fish.) Simmer, covered, 5 to 10 minutes or until fish flakes easily when tested with a fork. Remove fish to platter. Pour Lemon Butter Sauce over fish; garnish with parsley.

Lemon Butter Sauce: Melt butter; add lemon juice, stir to blend. Serve warm.

Nutrition per Serving
Carbs: 6 g Fiber: 2 g **Net Carbs: 4 g** Protein: 21 g Fat: 9 g Calories: 186

Entrées & Main Dishes, Fish/ Seafood

Sea Bass Palm Beach
Servings: 4

When I designed this recipe for the Country Club I advertised it as Low Carb, as I had a good number of members asking for Low Carb entrees. This was a huge success. You can eliminate the marjoram as I realize few people keep this in the pantry.
I have used other firm white fish for this recipe such as grouper. Any firm white fish will work fine. If you get a good buy on frozen fillets those will also work just fine for this recipe. Fortunately in S. Florida the fresh fish is plentiful.
I suggest serving this with a baby green salad with a simple vinaigrette.

2 pounds sea bass fillet, cut into 2" cubes
1/2 tablespoon olive oil
2 tablespoons onion, chopped
2 large tomatoes, diced
1 clove garlic, minced
1 tablespoon parsley, minced
1/4 teaspoon dried marjoram
1 whole bay leaf
1/2 cup dry red wine
1/2 cup heavy cream
1 tablespoon butter
1 tablespoon flour
Salt and pepper, to taste

Heat the oil in a large sauté pan, add onions, tomatoes, garlic, parsley and marjoram and cook gently for 5 minutes. Bury the bay leaf in the mixture and lay the sea bass chunks on top.
Mix the wine and cream together and pour over this mixture. Cover and cook in a 325 degree oven for 20 minutes.
Remove the sea bass to a serving platter, remove the veggies with a slotted spoon reserving the juice. Work the butter and flour together to form a paste, bring juice to a simmer and drop in this paste a little at a time and simmer to thicken, spoon over the sea bass and veggies and serve hot.

Nutrition per Serving
Carbs: 6 g Fiber: 1 g **Net Carbs: 5 g** Protein: 43 g Fat: 29 g Calories: 408

Entrées & Main Dishes, Fish & Seafood

Broiled Sea bass or New England Cod

Servings: 4

1 1/2 pounds Sea bass fillet or firm Cod
1 large tomato, sliced 1/2-inch thick
4 teaspoons fresh basil, finely chopped
4 teaspoons Parmesan cheese, grated
1/4 cup almonds, chopped
Salt and pepper (or to taste)
GARNISH
Lemon wedges
Parsley sprigs

Place fillets in an ovenproof pan. Coat the fillets lightly with olive oil and season with salt and pepper. Top each fillet with fresh basil and a tomato slice. Broil on high for approximately 10 minutes or until the tomatoes begin to brown. Mix almonds with cheese and sprinkle on each fillet. Broil a few minutes longer until nut mixture begins to brown. Garnish with parsley and lemon wedges.

Nutrition per Serving
Carbs: 3 g Fiber: 1 g **Net Carbs: 2 g** Protein: 3 g Fat: 5 g Calories: 67

Entrées & Main Dishes, Fish & Seafood

Red Snapper Vera Cruz

Servings: 4

1 pound snapper fillets boneless
2 tablespoons olive oil
1 small onion, thinly sliced
1/2 cup tomatoes, diced
1 bell pepper (red, green, or yellow), thinly sliced
3 cloves garlic, minced or pressed
1 teaspoon jalapeño or Serrano Chile (or to taste), chopped
1/2 teaspoon oregano
1 bay leaf
1/4 teaspoon salt and pepper
Juice of 2 lemons
1 lemon, sliced
GARNISH
Cilantro sprigs

Place red snapper fillets in shallow baking dish. Sauté onion, bell pepper, and garlic in olive oil until vegetables are limp. Add herbs, salt, pepper, tomatoes, and lemon juice. Pour this mixture over fish and arrange lemon slices over top. Cover tightly and bake at 325 degrees F for 25-30 minutes, just until fish turns opaque in center and begins to flake. During last 5 minutes, check for doneness and add liquid if needed. Continue to bake uncovered until fish is done.

Nutrition per Serving
Carbs: 6 g Fiber: 1 g **Net Carbs: 5 g** Protein: 24 g Fat: 8 g Calories: 195

Entrées & Main Dishes, Fish/ Seafood

Spicy Halibut with Creole Sauce
Servings: 4

Any other firm mild white fish can be used for this recipe. This is a fine example when using an IQF fillet would be perfect. Catfish is an excellent example of a fish to substitute.

2 pounds halibut, cut into 1" squares
Butter
1/2 cup onion, chopped
1 clove garlic, minced
3 tablespoons cooking oil
1/2 cup green bell pepper, chopped
1 bay leaf
1 cup whole tomato, chopped
1 teaspoon salt
1/8 teaspoon pepper
Tabasco to taste

Lightly grease a 9 × 9 baking dish with butter. Place cubed halibut in baking dish, cover and bake in a 350º degree oven for 20 minutes or until fish flakes easily with a fork.
While fish is baking, prepare the Creole sauce. Cook chopped onion and minced garlic clove in cooking oil until yellowed. Add chopped green pepper, bay leaf, whole tomatoes (cut into bite-sized pieces), season with salt and pepper. Simmer uncovered for 20 minutes. May add Tabasco, as desired. When fish is done, drain off excess liquid. Pour sauce over fish and serve hot.

Nutrition per Serving
Carbs: 5 g Fiber: 1 g **Net Carbs: 4 g** Protein: 48 g Fat: 16 g Calories: 63

Gregory Pryor C.E.C.

Entrées & Main Dishes, Fish & Seafood

Swordfish Piccata

Servings: 4

1 1/2 pounds swordfish, 4 1/2-inch thick steaks
1/2 teaspoon black pepper
4 tablespoons melted butter
2 teaspoons capers
2 tablespoons lemon juice
1 tablespoon parsley, finely chopped
GARNISH
Lemon rounds

Pepper Swordfish steaks and place in a broiling pan. Broil fish for 2 1/2 minutes on each side or until flesh turns opaque. Remove swordfish from broiling pan and place on a heated serving platter. Mix butter and lemon juice, add capers. Spoon over fish. Sprinkle with parsley. Garnish with lemon rounds.

Nutrition per Serving
Carbs: 1 g Fiber: 0 g **Net Carbs: 1 g** Protein: 34 g Fat: 7 g Calories: 209

Entrées & Main Dishes, Fish & Seafood

Tomato and Basil Flounder

Servings: 4

Two of my favorite flavors, tomato and basil come together as a sauce on this sautéed flounder dish. Try other herbs such as tarragon and chives in the place of the basil for an interesting twist.
For a nice plate presentation, place one fillet on a plate and top with vegetable mixture, chopped parsley and a sprig of fresh basil.
If flounder is not common to your region, any other firm mild white fish will work fine. I have even used fresh farm raised catfish fillets with great success.

4 whole roma tomato, diced
3 whole basil leaves
4 whole flounder fillets, boneless
2 tablespoons olive oil
1/2 cup onion, julienned
1 whole red pepper, julienned
2 tablespoons fresh rosemary, chopped
12 asparagus tips, blanched
Salt and pepper, to taste
Chopped parsley for garnish

Coat a large sauté pan with oil and heat over medium-high heat. Rinse fish in cold water and season with salt and pepper. Add fish to pan and sauté over medium heat. When done, remove fillets and keep warm. In the same pan, add onion and sauté until onions are translucent. Add peppers and cook an additional 2 minutes. Add tomatoes, rosemary and basil and season to taste with salt and pepper to taste. Cook for 10 minutes and add asparagus. A small amount of water or chicken stock may be needed to retain moisture. Cook another 5 minutes and serve.

Nutrition per Serving
Carbs: 10 g Fiber: 3 g **Net Carbs: 7 g** Protein: 33 g Fat: 9 g Calories: 253

Entrées & Main Dishes, Fish & Seafood

Shrimp Piccata
Servings: 4

Tiger Prawns are jumbo shrimp that are easily identifiable with the green stripe that runs every 1/4-inch across the tail. They are available in the seafood case at most grocery stores. However, feel free to substitute jumbo white or brown gulf shrimp in place of the tigers. Feel free to adjust the garlic or lemon in this recipe to suit your personal taste.
Although most feel that this has to be served over pasta, that's just not true. However if your Carb Count is low enough from the day, here is a perfect time to use the Low Carb Pasta. Otherwise simply thicken and serve in a bowl and enjoy the wonderful flavors with a crisp Caesar salad.

16 whole jumbo shrimp or tiger prawns
1/4 cup extra virgin olive oil
6 cloves garlic, sliced
1/4 cup shallots, minced
1/4 cup capers
1 tablespoon parsley, chopped fine
1 tablespoon basil leaf, chopped fine
1/4 cup lemon juice, fresh
1/4 cup dry white wine
1 cup fish stock
2 tablespoons ThickenThin®, or as needed

If you don't have any fish stock, take peelings from shrimp and place in 1 1/4 cups of water. Bring to a rolling boil, reduce to low and simmer 10-15 minutes. Strain and reserve. In a large mixing bowl, season shrimp to taste with salt and pepper. In a sauté pan, add oil over medium-high heat. Add garlic and sauté until edges begin to turn golden, then add shallots, Sauté 1 additional minute and add shrimp. Cook until pink and curled, approximately 2 minutes. Add capers, parsley, herbs, lemon juice and white wine. Bring to a simmer, reduce wine to 1/2 volume and add shrimp or fish stock. Bring to a simmer and cook. Add ThickenThin®. Season to taste using salt and pepper. When ready to serve, if serving Low Carb Pasta place hot pasta in the center of 4 serving dishes and top with the Piccata sauce and 4 jumbo shrimp.

Nutrition per Serving
Carbs: 6 g Fiber: 0 g **Net Carbs: 6 g** Protein: 6 g Fat: 15 g Calories: 204

Entrées & Main Dishes, Fish & Seafood

Shrimp Scampi
Servings: 4

Although scampi is a term used in some parts of the world to describe a certain species of shrimp, it is most often used to describe an Italian dish. This simple scampi recipe is magnificent when served over pasta, but in the Low Carb Lifestyle it may also be used as a topping for chicken and fish. Or how about a simple version of surf and turf, grill your favorite steak and top with or serve alongside for Low Carb Surf and Turf.

1 1/2 pounds fresh shrimp, 20-25 count peeled and deveined
1/4 cup extra virgin olive oil
6 cloves garlic, sliced
1/4 cup shallots, minced
1/4 cup mushrooms, sliced
1 tablespoon parsley, chopped fine
1 tablespoon basil leaf, chopped fine
1/4 cup dry white wine
2 tablespoons ThickenThin®, or as needed

Season shrimp lightly and set aside. In a large sauté pan, heat olive oil over medium-high heat. Add garlic and sauté 1-2 minutes or until edges turn golden. Add shrimp, shallots and basil. Using a slotted spoon, turn shrimp on each side until pink and curled. Add mushrooms, parsley and deglaze with white wine. Let wine come to a simmer and slightly reduce. Add ThickenThin® a little at a time to thicken as needed, or you can let the wine reduce till nearly evaporated and serve. Season to taste with salt and pepper.

Nutrition per Serving
Carbs: 5 g Fiber: 0 g **Net Carbs: 5 g** Protein: 35 g Fat: 16 g Calories: 9325

Gregory Pryor C.E.C.

Entrées & Main Dishes, Fish & Seafood

Curry Shrimp with Broccoli
Servings: 2

1/2 pound shrimp, peeled and deveined
4 tablespoons peanut oil
1/2 tablespoon soy sauce
1 cup broccoli flowerets, blanched
3 whole button mushrooms, quartered
1 tablespoon curry powder
5 tablespoons water, or as needed
1 tablespoon ThickenThin®

Blend 1 tablespoon of peanut oil and soy with shrimp to prevent them from sticking together during frying. In a wok or large skillet, heat 1 tablespoon peanut oil. Briefly stir-fry broccoli, and mushrooms. Remove and put in bowl and keep warm. Add an additional 2 tablespoons peanut oil to sauté pan or wok. Add shrimp and stir-fry to desired tenderness. Return vegetables to the pan or wok and sprinkle in the curry powder. Add a little water if needed. Taste the mixture and adjust seasonings or add more curry powder to you likening.
Thicken if needed with ThickenThin®.

Nutrition per Serving
Carbs: 10 g Fiber: 4 g **Net Carbs: 6 g** Protein: 27 g Fat: 30 g Calories: 407

Entrées & Main Dishes, Fish & Seafood

Cod Fillets Almandine

Servings: 4

You may use any other mild firm white fish for this recipe, however be certain the fillets are not more than 1/2 inch thick. The thicker fillets will require a longer cooking time and the almonds may burn.

4 whole cod fillets, boneless
2 whole eggs, beaten
1 tablespoon water
1/4 cup clarified butter
1 cup almond slivers, coarsely ground
Salt and pepper, to taste
2 tablespoons lemon juice

If fillets are large, cut into serving pieces. Season with 1 teaspoon salt and the pepper. Beat egg and water slightly. Dip fish into egg, then coat with almond flour. Add clarified butter to skillet; fry fish over medium-high heat about 10 minutes. Make certain to turn as needed to prevent the almond flour from burning. After fish is cooked, deglaze the pan with the lemon juice, scraping the pan and pour juice over fish.

Nutrition per Serving
Carbs: 8 g Fiber: 2 g **Net Carbs: 6 g** Protein: 51 g Fat: 36 g Calories: 549

Entrées & Main Dishes, Fish & Seafood

Blackened Dolphin, Grouper
Servings: 4

This is a versatile example of the simple process to making blackened fish.
It is best to use a heavy cast iron skillet and high heat. Be warned, if you do
not have a good overhead exhaust fan you will set off the smoke detectors.
Always choose the fish fillets that are 1/2 inch to 3/4 inch thick. Thicker
pieces will require finishing in a hot oven once the surface is blackened.
I have provided the formula for a blackening spice, however commercial
prepared versions are much easier and convenient to use.
I strongly recommend that you use clarified butter only, as using whole
butter will scorch or burn.

4 whole fish fillets
Blackening spice as needed
Clarified butter as needed, approx 1/2 cup.
Blackening spice as follows
2 tablespoons black pepper
2 tablespoons white pepper
1 tablespoon garlic powder
1 tablespoon thyme, dried
1 tablespoon dried parsley
2 tablespoons paprika
Combine all ingredients.

Pat each fillet dry with a paper towel. Pour the blackening spice into a pie pan or flat dinner plate and spread evenly. Heat the skillet over high heat. Dip each fillet in melted clarified butter then press into the spice and cover evenly. Place the fish in the hot skillet and cook till surface is nearly black. The side edges of the fillet will turn creamy white, this indicates the fish should be ready to turn and finish cooking. Serve hot with any side dish(s) of your choice.

Nutrition per Serving
Carbs: 7 g Fiber: 2 g **Net Carbs: 5 g** Protein: 42 g Fat: 2 g Calories: 218

Entrées & Main Dishes, Fish & Seafood

Simple Sautéed Fish Fillets

Servings: 4

This basic recipe works with absolutely ANY fish fillet. If your fillets are thinner than 3/4-inch, reduce the cooking time slightly. If they are thicker, increase the cooking time. When you have a great piece of fresh fish little is required to make it any better. This simple sauté is one of the easiest preparations you can use. The key here is having good quality fresh fish.
Spice up this basic recipe by adding 1 cup of cubed tomatoes and 1 chopped garlic clove to the pan before adding this fish. Let cook, stirring, for 2 minutes, then continue with the recipe.

4 whole fish fillets, boneless
1 tablespoon clarified butter
1 tablespoon olive oil
Salt and pepper, to taste
Lemon wedge and chopped parsley for garnish

Sprinkle the fish fillets with salt and pepper.
In a large skillet over medium-high heat, melt the butter and olive oil. Add the fish fillets and cook for about 2-3 minutes per side, or until it is just done. Fish is just done when you can press on the fillet and it flakes or separates.
Serve the fish immediately, garnished with the parsley and lemon wedges.

Nutrition per Serving
Carbs: 0 g Fiber: 0 g **Net Carbs: 0 g** Protein: 10 g Fat: 7 g Calories: 105

DESSERTS AND SWEETS

Without a doubt this is the one area of the Low Carb Lifestyle I am asked the most questions about. As we proceed about this topic my goal is to not just provide you with many rich rewarding desserts and sweets, but also to caution you on the excessive consumption of even our Low Carb versions. Why? Well simply inasmuch as we have made a decision to abandon the high carb sugar and starch habits of the past, simply replacing those with Low Carb acceptable sweets isn't always to our benefit. Remember before when I was explaining to you about how we have to train ourselves not to crave Carbs? Even though these recipes are well within the Low Carb range of a recipe, consuming sweets regularly is no more practical on a Low Carb Lifestyle that it was acceptable with your previous lifestyle. Even though before you weren't considering your daily Carbs as you are now, even then it was never acceptable to include sweets and desserts daily. My experience has proven to me that even consuming Low Carb desserts and sweet snack items in many people, further causes those cravings for sweets to grow or return once again.

Let me share with you a little something said to me when I was in Culinary College. It was during the pastry and desserts semester. We were in the kitchen making various types of "*puddings*" such as rice pudding, bread pudding etc. My instructor said to the class, *"if you intend to please the general American palate simply be certain your pudding is SWEET"*. Now think about that a minute. He didn't say make certain you use only quality products, nor did he say be certain to present the pudding in an appealing way. He said make certain it is sweet. Now what's the significance to this? Simple, Americans crave sweets. Sugar is one of those particular Carbs the body craves specifically. Satisfy that basic craving and you have temporarily stopped or reduced that craving for the time being. However, all you did was continue to give in to the craving till it appears again. And trust me, any or most of us know full well how serious that craving can be. Fortunately for myself I was never much of a sweets person even as a child. I rarely craved sweets in my younger years. In fact, even when I did crave sweets a small bowl of ice-cream or a piece of pie once a month was about as much as I ever had a craving for. However, having been in the food industry for many years I have seen firsthand the excessive amounts of sweets and desserts some people consume, often on a daily basis. My advice to you is this. If you were one of those people that ate sweets on a regular basis, but since changing to a Low Carb Lifestyle that urge has subsided I applaud you. I suggest you continue to minimize your sweets intake even the Low Carb versions, so as not to rekindle that habit or craving. If you're one of the many that still have those cravings after giving up typical high Carb desserts, I strongly recommend that you avoid from eating even the Low Carb versions till such time as that *"I have to have something sweet"* emotion is more under control. Although, for all the great many benefits of a Low Carb Lifestyle, other than weight loss and control, it is not a magic pill. It still requires you to be responsible. It requires you to make choices and to follow them for a Lifetime. And finally, it demands of you to break those high Carb habits and bonds.

These days at the Pryor family household it is just the two of us, my lovely wife and I. What I have been doing is making several different simple storable dessert items ahead of time in smaller portions and freezing these for those evenings when both of us just want something a little later in the evening. Although many of the dessert and sweets recipes I will provide to you will require a little extra effort than others, and some are best suited to be eaten within that day or two, we enjoy making some simple items such as mini cheese cakes that freeze so well. I make a 2 quart batch of Ice-Cream about once a month. It never last longer as my children even though now they know its Low Carb, always eat what we have when they stop over. Another favorite is Sugar-free Low Carb popsicles. I will explain these later. What you will not find in my recipes are concocted remakes of cakes and doughnuts made with ingredients you have to scour the planet for and pay huge sums of money for. Nor will you find any recipes that are some strange kitchen madman's blending of simply packaged sugar free mixes of who knows what. There are many Low Carb dessert and sweets we can make using natural Low Carb ingredients. That is what you will find in the sensible recipes provided in this book. Let me first share some guidelines for making a cheesecake. I have found that with the exception of Ice-Cream this is the most wholesome and rewarding of the Low Carb desserts. It is simple to make and stores wonderfully.

TIPS FOR THE PERFECT CHEESECAKE

Use these tips to create, bake, and store your perfect cheesecake. Bring all ingredients to room temperature before mixing. This usually takes thirty minutes. To soften cream cheese in the microwave; place unwrapped 8 oz. cheese in a microwavable bowl and microwave on high for 15 seconds. Add 15 seconds for each additional bar of cheese. Mix filling only until combined. Don't over mix. Use a spring form pan so the sides can be removed. Butter sides or use a metal spatula around the edges immediately after removing the cheesecake from the oven. Place spring form pan on a shallow pan, like a pizza pan, or cover bottom and up one inch around the sides with aluminum foil to avoid leaks in the oven. Place a shallow pan of water in rack below cheesecake to keep oven moist. Don't open oven door while baking. A perfectly baked cheesecake will be puffed around the edges. When shaken, about an inch in diameter in the center should jiggle. Cool slowly (about an hour) on a wire rack, away from any drafts. Store in the refrigerator, loosely covered, for up to four days. The bottom of the pan can be removed from the cheesecake once the cake has firmed in the refrigerator. Use two spatulas to move cake to serving platter. Garnishing a cheesecake should only be done within 1 to 3 hours of serving. Cheesecakes taste best when brought to room temperature. This takes about 30 minutes. Securely wrap an already firm, (about 4 hours in the refrigerator), cheesecake to be put in the freezer. Cheesecakes can be kept for up to 2 months in the freezer. Thaw frozen cheesecake overnight in the refrigerator. These guidelines will ensure you a rich creamy cheesecake. Few if any will ever suspect this of being Low Carb when using the recipe in this book. Fact is, for all practical purposes, all we do to make it a Low Carb cheesecake is replace the sugar with Splenda® and omit the flour, or any starch. I also use an extra egg or yolk to compensate for the lack of any starch.

Sweets

Basic Cheesecake
Servings: 8

This basic mix is wonderful just as is, but from this we can expand many flavors and types of cheesecakes. You can swirl some melted unsweet chocolate into the batter and mix with the tip of a knife to make a chocolate swirl cheesecake. If you choose this add an extra 1/8 cup Splenda®. Do not glaze this version with sour cream. By using Steels fruit fillings and topping you can make many varieties of fruit garnished cheesecakes.

24 ounces cream cheese, softened
3/4 cup Splenda®
1 tablespoon lemon juice
1 teaspoon lemon zest
1 1/2 teaspoons vanilla, divided
3 eggs
1 egg yolk
1 1/2 cups sour cream
3 tablespoons Splenda®

In a large bowl mix together softened cream cheese, Splenda® lemon juice, and zest. Make certain to mix well scraping down sides of bowl and beaters or paddle, removing any lumps. Add 1/2 tsp. vanilla, and eggs one egg at a time till well blended. Take care not to over mix the batter. Mix only till well blended.

Pour batter into either a nonstick spring form pan, or if using a silver type be certain to lightly butter the sides and bake in the center of the oven at 300 degree's for approx 55 to 60 minutes, or until the center is nearly set, but still jiggles in the center.

Remove from the oven, and mix the sour cream and remaining Splenda® and vanilla. Carefully spread this mixture evenly over the cake. Return to the oven and bake for 10 minutes.

Remove the cake, taking care to run a thin spatula or knife around the edge to loosen. Let cool well on a rack before removing the side. Refrigerate 4 hours or overnight.

Nutrition per Serving
Carbs: 5 g Fiber: 0 g **Net Carbs: 5 g** Protein: 10 g Fat: 40 g Calories: 417

Gregory Pryor C.E.C.

Chocolate Nut Clusters
Servings: 16

Store in container in refrigerator.
You may substitute any of the following ¼ cup hazelnut pieces chopped or
¼ cup macadamia nuts or ¼ cup chopped Brazil nuts.

4 ounces unsweetened baking chocolate, 4 squares
1/2 cup walnuts, pieces
1/4 cup pecan, pieces
1/2 cup unsalted butter, cut 1/2" thick
1/4 cup heavy cream
1 cup Splenda®
1 1/2 teaspoons vanilla extract
2 tablespoons shredded coconut meat, unsweetened

Place chocolate in 1 quart. Pyrex measuring cup and heat on high in microwave for one minute, stirring after 30 seconds. Add butter and heat for another 2-3 minutes, stirring every 30 seconds until chocolate and butter are melted. Add cream and whisk until blended. Add vanilla, nuts and Splenda®, blending rapidly while mixture is still warm.
Spread mixture on buttered dinner plate. Sprinkle with coconut. Cover with plastic wrap and freeze.
Remove from freezer and allow to warm up for 10-15 minutes. Break into 16 pieces.

Nutrition per Serving
Carbs: 3 g Fiber: 1 g **Net Carbs: 2 g** Protein: 2 g Fat: 15 g Calories: 139

Sweets

Lemon Curd

Servings: 4

3 egg yolks
1/4 cup Splenda®
1 1/2 teaspoons grated lemon rind
1/3 cup lemon juice
6 tablespoons unsalted butter

In heavy saucepan over medium heat combine yolks, Splenda® zest, juice and butter. Stir constantly 5-7 minutes until mixture coats the back of the spoon. Remove from heat and strain through a wire mesh sieve placed over a bowl. Place plastic wrap on surface of curd; refrigerate 1-hour or until cool.

Nutrition per Serving
Carbs: 2 g Fiber: 0 g **Net Carbs: 2 g** Protein: 2 g Fat: 21 g Calories: 203

Gregory Pryor C.E.C.

Ice-Cream

Chocolate Ice-Cream
Servings: 8

1 teaspoon gelatin
1 cup water
6 egg yolks
1 cup Splenda®
2/3 cup unsweetened cocoa
2 1/2 cups heavy cream
1 1/2 teaspoons vanilla extract
1 1/2 tablespoons chocolate extract

Sprinkle gelatin over water. Let stand until softened, at least 5 minutes.

In a medium bowl whisk yolks and Splenda® to combine. In a heavy saucepan mix gelatin mixture and cream. Add cocoa powder. Cook over medium-low heat, stirring occasionally, until cocoa is dissolved and mixture has begun to simmer.

Slowly pour one cup of gelatin cream mixture into yolk mixture to temper, whisking constantly. Pour yolk mixture back into the remaining mixture. Cook, stirring constantly, until mixture is thick enough to coat the back of a spoon.

Remove from heat. Stir in vanilla and chocolate extracts. Chill mixture 4 hours.

Pour ice-cream into ice-cream maker. Process according to manufacturer's directions.

Nutrition per Serving
Carbs: 6 g Fiber: 2 g **Net Carbs: 4 g** Protein: 5 g Fat: 32 g Calories: 331

Ice-Cream

Chocolate Pecan Ice-Cream

Servings: 8

1 tablespoon gelatin
1 cup water
6 egg yolks
1 cup Splenda®
2/3 cup unsweetened cocoa
2 1/2 cups heavy cream
1 1/2 teaspoons vanilla extract
1 1/2 teaspoons chocolate extract
1 cup pecans toasted, chopped

Sprinkle gelatin over water. Let stand until softened, at least 5 minutes.

In a medium bowl whisk yolks and Splenda® to combine. In a heavy saucepan mix gelatin mixture and cream. Add cocoa powder. Cook over medium low heat, stirring occasionally, until cocoa is dissolved and mixture has begun to simmer.

Slowly pour one cup of gelatin cream mixture into yolk mixture to temper, whisking constantly. Pour mixture back into the remaining mixture. Cook, stirring constantly, until mixture is thick enough to coat the back of a spoon.

Remove from heat. Stir in vanilla and chocolate extracts. Chill mixture 4 hours.

Process according to manufacturer's directions. Add chopped pecans 5 minutes before Ice-Cream is finished.

Nutrition per Serving
Carbs: 7 g Fiber: 2 g **Net Carbs: 5 g** Protein: 5 g Fat: 32 g Calories: 332

Gregory Pryor C.E.C.

Ice-Cream

Vanilla-Coconut Ice-Cream
Servings: 8

To toast coconut, spread evenly on a baking sheet and bake at 350° F for 5 minutes

6 egg yolks
3/4 cup Splenda®
2 cups heavy cream
1 can coconut milk unsweetened, 13.5 ounce can
2 teaspoons coconut extract
1 cup coconut meat, toasted, shredded

In a medium bowl whisk yolks and Splenda® to combine. In a heavy saucepan, bring heavy cream to a simmer over medium-low heat.
Slowly pour one cup cream into yolk mixture, whisking constantly. Pour yolk mixture back into saucepan. Cook, stirring constantly, until mixture is thick enough to coat the back of a spoon. Remove from heat. Stir in coconut milk, coconut and vanilla extracts. Chill 4 hours.
Pour ice-cream mix into ice-cream maker. Process according to manufacturer's directions. About 15 minutes before ice-cream is finished, add the toasted coconut.

Nutrition per Serving
Carbs: 3 g Fiber: 1 g **Net Carbs: 2 g** Protein: 4 g Fat: 29 g Calories: 285

Sweets

Chilled Zabaglione
Servings: 4

For a different version, omit the Marsala wine and substitute champagne.

6 tablespoons Splenda®
1 teaspoon unflavored gelatin
1/2 cup Marsala wine
6 egg yolks, beaten until thick
1 cup whipping cream
1 teaspoon vanilla extract
4 egg whites
1/8 teaspoon salt
1/8 teaspoon cream of tartar
Fresh strawberries or raspberries (Optional)

In double boiler, combine 4 tablespoons Splenda® and gelatin. Add Marsala wine and beaten egg yolks. Cook over hot water, stirring constantly, until mixture thickens. Remove from heat and chill until cool but not set.
In a chilled medium bowl, whip cream and vanilla until stiff. Add chilled egg yolk mixture to cream and beat until smooth.
In another bowl, beat egg whites until foamy. Add salt, cream of tartar and 2 tablespoons Splenda®; beat until stiff peaks form. Fold beaten egg whites into cream mixture. Spoon into dessert glasses. Chill. Serve with berries. (Optional)

Nutrition per Serving
Carbs: 4 g Fiber: 0 g **Net Carbs: 4 g** Protein: 9 g Fat: 30 g Calories: 339.

Gregory Pryor C.E.C.

Sweets

Almond Pound Cake
Servings: 8

Some variations are: Add cocoa and eliminate lemon extract for chocolate pound cake. Add banana extract instead of lemon and some chopped nuts for a banana nut cake.

1 cup unsalted butter
1 cup Splenda®
5 whole eggs
2 cups almond flour, ground
1 teaspoon baking powder
1 teaspoon lemon extract
1 teaspoon vanilla extract

Preheat oven to 350°F.
Cream butter and Splenda®. Add eggs, one at a time, beating after each.
Mix almond flour with baking powder; add to egg mixture a little at a time.
Add extracts.
Pour into 9" greased cake pan. Bake for 50-55 minutes.

Nutrition per Serving
Carbs: 7 g Fiber: 2 g **Net Carbs: 5 g** Protein: 11 g Fat: 45 g Calories: 459

Sweets

Sponge Cake

Servings: 9

5 whole eggs, separated
1 1/2 tablespoons vanilla extract
3 tablespoons cake flour
1/2 teaspoon cream of tartar
5 tablespoons Splenda®
1 teaspoon lemon juice
4 tablespoons heavy cream

Place egg yolks and Splenda® in a bowl. Beat till yolks are fluffy and pale yellow. Add vanilla extract and lemon juice. Continue to beat and add cake flour one tablespoon at a time. Stir in heavy cream. Beat egg whites in fresh bowl with cream of tartar until stiff but not dry. Fold yolk mixture into egg whites. Be careful not to break down egg whites, fold carefully and slowly. Turn into greased 9" cake pan and bake at 325°F for 30 minutes or until cake tests done. Inserted tooth pick comes out clean.

Nutrition per Serving
Carbs: 3 g Fiber: 0 g **Net Carbs: 3 g** Protein: 3 g Fat: 5 g Calories: 74

Gregory Pryor C.E.C.

Sweets

Pumpkin Pie

Servings: 8

2/3 cup soy flour
1/3 cup almonds, toasted, chopped
1/3 cup whole grain flour
1/4 cup Splenda®
6 tablespoons butter, unsalted, cut into 1" cubes
2 tablespoons ice water
1 can pumpkin puree, 15 ounce can
1/2 cup Splenda®
1 teaspoon ground cinnamon
3/4 teaspoon ground ginger
1/4 teaspoon ground clove
1/4 teaspoon salt
2 large eggs
1 1/4 cups heavy cream

Heat oven to 425°F. In a large bowl whisk together soy flour, almonds, whole grain flour and Splenda®. Cut in butter with a pastry blender or two knives until butter pieces are about the size of peas. Add the ice water a little at a time; stir to combine. (You may have to add more or less water depending on the absorption of the mix).

Transfer crust mixture to a 9" pie pan. Press along bottom and sides of pie pan to shape the crust. Place in freezer to firm, about 20 minutes.

Cover crust loosely with aluminum foil and bake 15 minutes; remove from oven and take off foil. Reduce oven to 375°F.

In a bowl, whisk pumpkin, Splenda®, cinnamon, ginger, cloves, and salt to combine. Mix in eggs, one at a time.

Add heavy cream and mix well. Pour filling into partially baked piecrust. Cover crust edge with aluminum foil. Bake 40 minutes, or until filling is set but the center still jiggles when shaken. Cool on a wire rack.

Nutrition per Serving
Carbs: 12 g Fiber: 3 g **Net Carbs: 9 g** Protein: 7 g Fat: 28 g Calories: 318

Sweets

Pecan Pie
Servings: 8

Several years ago I was asked by the Atkins's group to create a Low Carb Thanksgiving menu. This was one of the featured recipes. I have slightly revised it since then. Most larger supermarkets now carry Atkins brand pancake syrup. This is the syrup I use in this recipe.
Pie may be refrigerated for up to 3 days. Reheat in a warm oven before serving.

Crust
1/2 cup almond flour
1/4 cup flour, all-purpose
1 tablespoon Splenda®.
1/2 stick butter
Filling
1 1/2 cups sugar free pancake syrup, see note
4 whole eggs
1/2 cup Splenda®
5 tablespoons butter, melted
1 teaspoon vanilla extract
1 piece salt
2 cups pecan halves, toasted

Heat oven to 350ºF. Mix almond flour, all-purpose flour and Splenda® in a large bowl. Stir in butter with a fork. Chill crumb mixture 20 minutes. With your fingertips press crumb mixture on bottom and sides of a 9" pie plate. Bake 7 minutes, until browned and set. Remove from oven; cool. Increase oven temperature to 375ºF.

For filling, bring syrup to a simmer in a small saucepan. Cook 10 minutes, until reduced by half. Remove from heat; cool to room temperature.

In a large bowl, whisk eggs, Splenda® melted butter and extract. Whisk in syrup. Add toasted pecans and combine well. Pour mixture into prepared piecrust and bake 20 minutes until edges are firm (center will be quivery). Transfer to a wire rack to cool.

Nutrition per Serving
Carbs: 10 g Fiber: 3 g **Net Carbs: 7 g** Protein: 7 g Fat: 38 g Calories: 396.

Gregory Pryor C.E.C.

Sweets

Peanut Butter Cookies
Servings: 16

1/2 cup chunky peanut butter (sugar free) I prefer the natural
3/4 cup Heavy Cream
1 egg yolk
1/4 cup Chopped Macadamia Nuts Chopped fine (optional)
2 tsp. vanilla extract
4 tablespoons Splenda®
2 Tbs. all-purpose flour
Pinch of salt

Preheat an oven to 375. Spray a cookie sheet with Pam or other pan release no carb spray.

Mix all ingredients in a bowl till well mixed. Chill ingredients for 10 minutes. Roll tsp. size balls of dough and place on sheet pan, slightly indent each with the back of a fork, or drop on sheet pan with a teaspoon.

Bake about 10-12 minutes or until slightly brown.

Nutrition per Serving
Carbs: 3 g Fiber: 1 g **Net Carbs: 2 g** Protein: 4 g Fat: 5 g Calories: 52

Sweets

Shortbread Cookies
Servings: 16

1 cup Almond flour
1/4 cup all-purpose flour
1 cup Splenda®
1 whole egg
1 egg yolk
1 tsp. vanilla extract
¼ cup softened butter
Sugar free fruit preserve (optional as needed)

Preheat oven to 350. Mix almond flour, A-P flour and Splenda®. In a separate bowl beat egg and egg yolk, add vanilla and butter and mix till incorporated. Add this to the dry ingredients and mix well.

Form 24 small balls and place on a cookie sheet. Lightly flatten to silver dollar size. Bake for approximately 8 to 10 minutes. Cool before service.

Fruit filling option; after lightly flattening cookie, lightly indent with the back of a tablespoon or use your thumb a small indentation in the center of each cookie. Fill this with the sugar free preserve of choice. I prefer raspberry.

Nutrition per Serving
Carbs: 3 g Fiber: 1 g **Net Carbs: 3 g** Protein: 5 g Fat: 6 g Calories: 52

Gregory Pryor C.E.C.

Sweets

Macaroon Cookies
Servings: 16

1/2 cup heavy cream
4 tablespoons Splenda®
1/4 teaspoon vanilla extract
1/4 teaspoon almond extract
1 cup shredded coconut meat, unsweetened
2 whole egg whites
1 pinch cream of tartar
1 pinch salt

Mix cream with sweetener and extracts. Add coconut and mix well. Let stand for 1-hour. If mixture feels dry to the touch after 1-hour, add a little more cream.
Preheat oven to 350°F.
Whip egg whites until peaks form. Fold into coconut. Using a teaspoon, place a small amount of coconut mix onto a well greased cookie sheet, repeating to make approximately 16 cookies. Bake until slightly browned (usually 12-15 minutes). If tops have not browned in 15 minutes, you can place them under the broiler for a few minutes (watch them carefully!) Allow to cool before serving.

Nutrition per Serving
Carbs: 2 g Fiber: 1 g **Net Carbs: 1 g** Protein: 4 g Fat: 4 g Calories: 46
For a chocolate version of this recipe, omit the almond extract and add 3 tablespoons of unsweetened Cocoa Powder with the cream and coconut mixture. Proceed with recipe. Add 1 gram extra Carb to the net.

Sweets

Sugar Cookies
Servings: 24

This is one of the five different Low Carb cookies I developed for a national food show. Few people ever considered these to be Low Carb.
There is a little trick to creating the Almond flour for cookies. You must have fine smooth flour, for all but the peanut butter version. To make the flour smooth, process in a food processor using a pulsed action to break down the almonds, then let this cool in the bowl a few minutes. Process again until the flour is very fine. The heat from the food processor action can cause this to become like a paste.
Second trick. Make a powdered sugar likeness using this same technique with Splenda®. Process till very fine.

1 1/4 cups almond flour
1 cup Splenda®
1 whole egg
1 whole egg yolk
1 teaspoon vanilla extract
1/4 cup unsalted butter

Preheat oven to 350°F.
Mix almond flour with Splenda®, sifting until well mixed. In a separate bowl, lightly beat egg and then mix well with extracts and softened butter. Add to dry ingredients and mix well.
Form dough into 24 small balls and space evenly on two ungreased cookie sheets. Press moderately to flatten to a silver-dollar pancake size. If you choose, sprinkle liberally with fine processed Splenda®, just as you would traditional sugar cookies. Bake for approximately 8 minutes at 350°. They will slide right off the cookie sheet. Cool 5 minutes before eating.

Nutrition per Serving
Carbs: 1 g Fiber: trace g **Net Carbs: 1 g** Protein: 2 g Fat: 6 g Calories: 67

Gregory Pryor C.E.C.

Sweets

Fudge
Servings: 24

If you follow this recipe exactly as it is written you will marvel at the quality of the fudge. No one will ever believe this is Low Carb.

3 cups Splenda®
1/2 cup butter
1 cup whole milk
1 pinch Salt
4 ounces unsweetened baking chocolate
1 teaspoon vanilla extract
1 cup walnuts, chopped

Butter an 8 x 8-inch pan. Combine Splenda®, butter, milk, salt, and chocolate in medium saucepan. Stirring constantly, cook over medium heat until all ingredients melt and come to a boil. Do not scrape down the sides of the pan. Lower heat, insert candy thermometer, and let boil slowly without stirring for about 10 minutes or until soft ball forms when dropped in a cup of cold water (238 degrees F on a candy thermometer). Remove pan from heat and cool. (Important note, the mixture should be very cool, almost near body temperature before agitating the mixture. Failure to do so will result in a *"grainy"* product. Add vanilla. Beat steadily until fudge loses its gloss. Add nuts. Pour into pan. Cool for 20 minutes and cut into squares. Store in airtight container or wrap in foil.

Nutrition per Serving
Carbs: 2 g Fiber: 1 g **Net Carbs: 1 g** Protein: 2 g Fat: 10 g Calories: 97

The following recipe is a bit tricky. I suggest you familiarize yourself completely before taking on this recipe. Although it has been, and continues to be, my intent to provide you with as simple a recipe as possible, when we create dessert recipes, often the techniques we must use to keep the Low Carb count of a recipe requires us to use specific techniques. One of which is to replace bakers chocolate in the following recipes. By using the following technique we reduce the net Carbs drastically. As much as I recommend not using partially hydrogenated fats, for this procedure we must use a small amount of shortening. To replicate the Bakers chocolate we would normally use in these recipes we will use the table that follows. I recommend only using Dutch Cocoa for this recipe, as the flavor, color and quality is unsurpassed compared to standard Cocoa powder.

"Dutching" is a process in which unsweetened cocoa powder is mixed with an alkalizing agent to neutralize the natural acidity of cocoa. This process gives. Dutch Processed Cocoa a milder, mellower flavor and a darker, richer color than traditional Cocoa. For those reasons, the flavor and color of *"Dutched"* cocoa is often desired in gourmet recipes. Use Dutch Processed Cocoa for the following substitutions. For each ounce of Bakers Chocolate called for in the recipe use the following equation:

Substitutions

Cocoa can be used as an easy substitute for most forms of baking chocolate and even baking chips called for in recipes. Use the following chart as a guideline for your needs:

Product	Cocoa	Shortening	Splenda®.	Amount
Unsweetened Baking Chocolate Premelted	3 Tbsp.	1 Tbsp.		Equals 1 oz. Scale up accordingly.
Unsweetened Baking Chocolate	3 Tbsp.	1 Tbsp.		Equals 1 envelope
Semi-Sweet Baking Chocolate	6 Tbsp.	1/4 cup	7 Tbsp.	Equals 6 oz. Semi-Sweet Baking Chocolate or 1 cup Semi-Sweet Chocolate Chips
Sweet Baking Chocolate	3 Tbsp.	2-2/3 Tbsp.	4-1/2 Tbsp.	Equals 4 oz bar

Combine the shortening, Cocoa and if called for Splenda®. And proceed with the recipe using this substitution in place of the Bakers Chocolate.

As I indicated previously, this recipe in particular may seem a bit complicated. In truth if you have the basic baking skills to make a cake, you can prepare this recipe will equal success.

Sweets

Flourless Sheet Cake
Servings: 12

To make the filling for this recipe, in a chilled mixing bowl on medium speed whip one cup of heavy cream until soft peaks appear. Continue to whip adding 2 tablespoons Splenda®. Whip until firm. Should you enjoy a coffee flavored filling, add 2 teaspoons instant coffee or to taste to the cream. Another flavorful example would be to use Steels Low Carb fruit filling in place of the whipped cream. Just remember to figure in the Cabs for the amount of filling you use.
By using the Cocoa conversion the net Carbs are reduced to net 5g.

6 ounces semisweet chocolate, see substitution table
3 tablespoons coffee, strong flavored coffee
1 teaspoon vanilla extract
6 large egg whites
1/4 teaspoon cream of tartar
3/4 cup Splenda®
6 large egg yolks, beaten
2 cups whipped cream, see directions

Have all ingredients at room temperature. Preheat the oven to 375 degrees. Lightly grease a 17 1/2 by 11 1/2 baking sheet pan (jelly roll pan) and line bottom with wax or parchment paper. In a medium heat proof bowl combine the chocolate, coffee and vanilla. Set the bowl in a large skillet of simmering water and stir often, until the chocolate is melted and the mixture is smooth but not hot. Remove from the heat. In a large clean bowl on medium speed, beat the egg whites until soft peaks form. Add the cream of tarter and continue to beat, adding the Splenda®, a little at a time. Beat whites until peaks are stiff but not dry. Whisk into the chocolate mixture the 6 egg yolks.

Carefully using a rubber spatula fold into the chocolate mixture 1/3 of the whites. Add this back into the egg whites and fold together. Scrape the batter into the prepared baking pan and spread evenly. Bake in the center of the oven for 10 minutes, and then reduce the temperature to 350 and bake until the top is firm to the touch, 5 - 7 minutes longer. Remove from the oven and let the cake cool in the pan on a cooling rack. The cake will sink as it cools. Do not be alarmed should the cake have cracks, this is normal. Once the cake is completely cooled, run a thin knife along the edges to release the cake. Invert the cake onto a large sheet of aluminum foil.

Peel of the paper. Spread the whipped cream evenly over the cake. Gently roll the cake in a jelly roll fashion.

Refrigerate at least one hour before slicing into 12 servings. Or slice the number of servings needed. Cover with plastic wrap and store in the refrigerator.

Nutrition per Serving
Carbs: 5 g Fiber: 0 g **Net Carbs: 5 g** Protein: 4 g Fat: 14 g Calories: 176

In concluding the dessert section of this book let me suggest a few simple and easy (*no recipe needed*) ideas. Earlier I mentioned making popsicles; yes I know this doesn't sound very elegant. However oftentimes having these in the freezer is just what we might want as the evening comes to a close and that something cold and sweet desire overcomes you. To make these in solid or multicolored is simple. First you of course will need some Popsicle molds and sticks. These are commonly found in most discount stores such as Wal-Mart. I bought mine from the local Bed Bath and Beyond. They had a nice set on sale. I use Crystal Light® drink mix. Simply fill and freeze. To make multicolored popsicles mix several flavors as chosen, partially fill and partially freeze each flavor. Once the first flavor is set add the next and continue till the molds are full. Another easy and Low Carb treat to keep is the sugar free Jello and Jello brand pudding cups. As I stated earlier in this book, the new additions to Low Carb products is growing weekly, so every time your at the supermarket, browse the isles checking the labels of the many products that might appeal to you that you may not have considered would be Low carb. So many products are suitable for our Low Carb Lifestyle; we just have to be diligent in our shopping.

RECIPE MAKE OVER

Now let's take a look at a few made over recipes. I have chosen two random recipes that should clearly demonstrate how we first recognize the High Carb ingredients, and how, with a few simple revisions we can revise the recipe to conform to a Low Carb Plan. Not only did I reduce the net Carbs, I also, in my opinion made the recipes more flavorful and practical. When we look at any recipe, it is often simple to spot the High Carb offenders. Specifically the more you become accustomed to thinking Low Carb and develop the awareness of the High Carb presence that most recipes include. Many times we have to omit an ingredient, whereas other times, often simply reducing the quantity and adding another Low Carb ingredient to compensate for the total volume of the recipe is all that is required. When you look at the following examples, I have altered the text on the original recipe to point out the areas where we can make the revisions to lower the net Carbs.

Let's take a look now and examine the reasons I have changed each as I have.

Mashed Potato Chicken Casserole

Servings: 6

2 cups cooked cubed chicken
1 jar Chicken Tonight Cooking Sauce for Chicken—Creamy Mushroom
1 10-ounce package frozen baby carrots
1 cup frozen peas
1 tablespoon chopped fresh parsley
1/2 teaspoon salt
Pinch black pepper
1 cup shredded Cheddar cheese
4 cups prepared instant mashed potatoes, prepared according to package directions

Preheat oven to 350 degrees F.
In a large skillet, combine cooked chicken with sauce. Simmer over low heat 5 minutes or until heated through. Add carrots, peas, parsley, salt and pepper. Heat thoroughly 10 minutes, stirring frequently. Spoon chicken mixture into a 2 1/2 quart casserole dish. Evenly top with Cheddar cheese. Spoon mashed potatoes over casserole. Bake 30 minutes, or until bubbly and potatoes are lightly browned.

Nutrition per Serving
Carbs: 35 g Fiber: 5 g **Net Carbs: 30 g** Protein: 10 g Fat: 12.5 g Calories: 320

Mashed Potato Chicken Casserole (Low Carb)

Servings: 6

2 cups cooked cubed chicken
1 cup Low Carb Mushroom Sauce
1 cup broccoli florets, blanched
1/2 cup cauliflower flowerets, blanched
1 tablespoon chopped fresh parsley
1/2 teaspoon salt
Pinch black pepper
1 cup shredded Cheddar cheese
3 cups Mock Mashed Potatoes
2 tablespoons clarified butter

Preheat oven to 350 degrees F.
In a large skillet, combine cooked chicken with sauce. Simmer over low heat 5 minutes or until heated through. Add broccoli, cauliflower, parsley, salt and pepper. Heat thoroughly 10 minutes, stirring frequently. Spoon chicken mixture into a 2 1/2 quart casserole dish. Evenly top with Cheddar cheese. Spoon mock mashed potatoes over casserole, drizzle clarified butter over top. Bake 30 minutes, or until bubbly and potatoes are lightly browned.

Nutrition per Serving
Carbs: 11 g Fiber: 3 g **Net Carbs: 8 g** Protein: 19 g Fat: 12.5 g Calories: 379

First let's review the recipe on the left. The first suspect ingredient is the prepared mushroom sauce. From experience we know that typical commercially prepared sauces are full of starch, sugars and in most white sauces, whole milk solids, another high Carb ingredient. Obviously using our own Low Carb sauce in this case in and of its self, omits a large number of Carbs. Second the flavor of our own prepared sauce is much more flavorful. Next we see one package of carrots. This is always a trouble spot, as carrots are high in Carbs. The solution for this example is simple; replace the carrots with a Low Carb high fiber vegetable. In this example, broccoli. Next, another of those High Carb vegetables are the Peas. Again we have to replace these with a better choice, in this example cauliflower. Now as you review these changes, other than Carbs we have not given up anything at all. In fact I think we have improved this recipe, both in flavor, texture and most importantly Carb reduction. Finally the mashed potatoes. Well this is a no brainer. Instant potatoes in its self, are just not good, period. They taste instant, feel instant and are high in Carbs. The revision to this ingredient is simple and obvious. Now we have a recipe that was once one we could not even consider preparing, to one that is well within the Low Carb plan. Reducing from 30g of Carbs, to a manageable 8g. Now let's look at another with fewer ingredients, yet, one we can easily revise to fit our Lifestyle.

Gregory Pryor C.E.C.

Pollock Chowder
Servings: 6

1 1/2 pounds Alaska Pollock fillets, thawed if necessary
1 cup onion, chopped
1/2 cup celery, sliced
1 clove garlic, minced
1 tablespoon oil
2 14 1/2-ounce cans tomatoes (14 1/2 to 16-ounce cans)
3/4 cup water
1/4 cup dry white wine
OR
1/4 cup water
1/2 teaspoon oregano, crushed
1/2 teaspoon salt
1/8 teaspoon pepper
Dash bottled hot pepper sauce

Cut Alaska Pollock into large chunks.
Sauté onion, celery and garlic in oil. Add tomatoes including liquid, water, wine and seasonings. Bring to boil; simmer 10 minutes. Add Alaska Pollock; simmer, covered, about 10 minutes or until fish flakes when tested with a fork.

Nutrition per Serving
Carbs: 12 g Fiber: 1 g **Net Carbs: 11 g** Protein: 21 g Fat: 3 g Calories: 167.

Pollock Chowder (Low Carb)
Servings: 6

1 1/2 pounds Alaska Pollock fillets, thawed if necessary
1/2 cup onion, chopped
1/2 cup celery, sliced
1 clove garlic, minced
1 tablespoon oil
2 large tomatoes, diced
3/4 cup chicken stock
1/4 cup dry white wine
OR
1/4 cup water
1/2 teaspoon oregano, crushed
1/2 teaspoon salt
1/8 teaspoon pepper
Dash bottled hot pepper sauce

Cut Alaska Pollock into large chunks.
Sauté onion, celery and garlic in oil. Add tomatoes including liquid, stock, wine and seasonings. Bring to boil; simmer 10 minutes. Add Alaska Pollock; simmer, covered, about 10 minutes or until fish flakes when tested with a fork.

Nutrition per Serving
Carbs: 4 g Fiber: 1 g **Net Carbs: 3 g** Protein: 20 g Fat: 3 g Calories: 138

Once again, first reviewing the recipe on the left. Onions as we know are high in Carbs, as they contain a fairly large amount of sugar. For this reason onions are often used in a recipe so that as they are sweated they release their sugar and add some tender sweetness to a recipe. So our first task is to decide, does this particular dish really require this amount of onions. The answer is no. We will improve the overall flavor as we continue to make our revisions. So in this example we decrease the amount of the high Carb onions. Second in the list is a true offender; canned tomatoes. Commercially prepared canned tomatoes have a significant amount of added sugar to preserve the tomatoes for canning. Secondly, the tomatoes used for canning are hothouse tomatoes that would be bland and nearly flavorless if not for the added ingredients used in canning. Tomatoes naturally have some sugar content which when used fresh in proper amounts are an acceptable Low Carb item. Finally when we substitute fresh for canned we are not losing a significant amount of tomato volume at all. If you were to drain a 14 oz. can of tomatoes, you would clearly see the yield of tomato would be less than the yield of one large fresh tomato, just as we have substituted in this recipe. Finally, and for the life of me, I never understand why so many recipes call for water as part of the cooking liquid that becomes part of the sauce. Water is flavorless. So, we replace the water in this recipe with chicken stock. Now the final result; we have omitted a significant number of Carbs as well as enhanced the flavor of the dish. Even if you don't have homemade stock, using canned chicken broth in this case would be a better choice than water. I will share a fact with you. When I am preparing almost any recipe, I always use stock in place of water. If I am blanching vegetables, I use stock. Not only does the stock add flavor to the vegetables, now I also have an even better flavored stock after the vegetables are blanched or cooked to use at another time. This same reserved stock is simply strained and stored for later use, often times I label this stock for making soups.

I sincerely wish this book has inspired you to believe in the Low Carb Lifestyle, as being the final dietary change you will ever have to make. As well as enjoy the health and rewards associated with this Lifestyle. It has been the most intelligent decision I have ever made about my health. Further it has improved the quality of life that I have come to appreciate from this responsible Lifestyle.

God Bless and Bon Appetite'.

COMMON COOKING TERMS

AERATE

To pass dry ingredients through a fine-mesh sifter so large pieces can be removed. The process also incorporates air to make ingredients like flour, lighter. Sifting dry ingredients aerates them while distributing small amounts of chemical leaveners or dry seasoning evenly through the mixture. Use sifters, sieves or tamis to both aerate and sift.

BARD

To tie fat around lean meats or fowl to keep them from drying out during roasting. The fat bastes the meat while it cooks, keeping it moist and adding flavor. The fat is removed a few minutes before the meat is finished, allowing the meat to brown. Barding is necessary only when there is no natural fat present.

BASTE

To brush or spoon food as it cooks with melted fat or the cooking juices from the dish. Basting prevents foods from drying out and adds color and flavor.

Gregory Pryor C.E.C.

BLANCH

To cook raw ingredients in boiling water briefly. Blanched vegetables are generally "*shocked*" i.e. plunged immediately and briefly into an ice water bath to stop the cooking process and preserve color and crunch.

BLEND

To combine two or more ingredients together with a spoon, beater or blender.

BOIL

To heat a liquid to its boiling point, until bubbles break the surface. "*Boil*" also means to cook food in a boiling liquid.

BONE

To remove the bones from meat, fish or fowl. Use a sharp boning knife and angle the blade toward the bone to avoid tearing or nicking the flesh.

BRAISE

To cook food, tightly covered, in a small amount of liquid at low heat for a long period of time. Sometimes, the food is first browned in fat. The long, slow cooking tenderizes meats by gently breaking down their fibers. The braising liquid keeps meats moist and can be used as a basis for sauce. Use wine, stocks or water as components in braising liquid.

BROIL

To cook food directly above or under a heat source. Food can be broiled in an oven or on a grill.

BRUSH

To apply a liquid, like a glaze, to the surface of food using a pastry brush.

BUTTERFLY

To split food (meat, fish, fowl) down the center, cutting almost, but not completely through. The two halves are then opened flat to resemble a butterfly.

CANNEL

To create small V-shaped grooves over the surface of fruits or vegetables for decorative purposes using a canelle knife. The fruit or vegetable is then sliced, creating a decorative border on the slices.

CARAMELIZE

To heat sugar until it liquefies and become a clear caramel syrup ranging in color from golden to dark brown. Fruits and vegetables with natural sugars can be caramelized by sautéing, roasting or grilling, giving them a sweet flavor and golden glaze.

CHIFFONADE

To slice into very thin strips or shreds. Literally translated from French, the term means *"made of rags"*.

CHOP

To cut food into bite-size pieces using a knife. A food processor may also be used to chop food. Chopped food is more coarsely cut than minced food.

CLARIFY

To remove sediment from a cloudy liquid, thereby making it clear. To clarify liquids, such as stock, egg whites and/or eggshells are commonly added and simmered for approximately 15 minutes. The egg whites attract and trap particles from the liquid. After cooling, strain the mixture through a cloth-lined sieve to remove residue. To clarify rendered fat, add hot water and boil for about 15 minutes. The mixture should then be strained through several layers of cheesecloth and chilled. The resulting layer of fat should be completely clear of residue.

Clarified butter is butter that has been heated slowly so that its milk solids separate and sink, and can be discarded. The resulting clear liquid can be used at a higher cooking temperature and will not go rancid as quickly as un-clarified butter.

CURE

To treat food by one of several methods for preservation purposes. Examples are smoking, pickling – in an acid base, corning – with acid and salt, and salt curing – which removes water.

DEEP-FRY

To cook food in hot fat or oil deep enough so that it is completely covered. The temperature of the fat is extremely important and can make the difference between success and failure. When the fat is not hot enough, the food absorbs fat and becomes greasy. When the fat is too hot, the food burns on the exterior before it has cooked through. Fat at the correct temperature will produce food with a crisp, dry exterior and moist interior. An average fat temperature for deep-frying is 375 degrees, but the temperature varies according to the food being fried. Use a deep fryer, an electric fry pan or a heavy pot and a good kitchen thermometer for deep frying.

DEGLAZE

To remove browned bits of food from the bottom of a pan after sautéing, usually meat. After the food and excess fat have been removed from the pan, a small amount of liquid is heated with the cooking juices in the pan and stirred to remove browned bits of food from the bottom. The resulting mixture often becomes the base for a sauce.

DEGORGE

1. To sprinkle vegetables with salt to eliminate water. Eggplant for example are generally salted and patted dry before cooking.
2. To add cornmeal to water and soak crustaceans in order that they will eliminate the sand in their shells.

DEVEIN

To remove the blackish-gray vein from the back of a shrimp. The vein can be removed with a special utensil called a deveiner or with the tip of a sharp knife. Small and medium shrimp need deveining for aesthetic purposes only. However, because the veins in large shrimp contain grit, they should always be removed.

DICE

To cut food into tiny cubes (about 1/8- to 1/4-inch).

DRAIN

To pour off fat or liquid from food, often using a colander.

DREDGE

To lightly coat food that is going to be fried with flour, ground nuts, breadcrumbs or cornmeal. The coating helps to brown the food and provides a crunchy surface. Dredged foods need to be cooked immediately, while breaded foods, those dredged in flour, dipped in egg then dredged again in breading, can be prepared and held before cooking.

EMULSIFY

To bind together two liquid ingredients that normally do not combine smoothly, such as water and fat. Slowly add one ingredient to the other while mixing rapidly. This action disperses tiny droplets of one liquid in the other. Mayonnaise and vinaigrettes are emulsions. Use a good whisk for steady, even emulsification.

FILLET

To create a fillet of fish or meat by cutting away the bones. Fish and boning knives help produce clean fillets.

FOLD

To combine a light mixture like beaten egg whites with a much heavier mixture like whipped cream. In a large bowl, place the lighter mixture on top of the heavier one. Starting at the back of the bowl, using the edge of a rubber spatula, cut down through the middle of both mixtures, across the bottom of the bowl and up the near side. Rotate the bowl a quarter turn and repeat. This process gently combines the two mixtures.

FRY

To cook food (non-submerged) in hot fat or oil over moderate to high heat. There is very little difference between frying and SAUTÉING although sautéing is often thought of as being faster and using less fat.

GRATE

To reduce a large piece of food to coarse or fine threads by rubbing it against a rough, serrated surface, usually on a grater. A food processor, fitted with the appropriate blades, can also be used for grating. The food that is being grated should be firm. Cheese that needs to be grated can be refrigerated first for easier grating.

GRILL

To cook food on a grill over hot coals or other heat source. The intense heat creates a crust on the surface of the food which seals in the juices. The grill should be clean and must be heated before the food is laid on it. The food can also be basted and seasoned.

GRIND

To reduce food to small pieces by running it through a grinder. Food can be ground to different degrees, from fine to coarse.

HOMOGENIZE

To create an emulsion by reducing all the particles to the same size. The fat globules are broken down mechanically until they are evenly distributed throughout the liquid. Homogenized milk and some commercial salad dressings are two examples of homogenized foods.

INFUSE

To steep an aromatic ingredient in hot liquid until the flavor has been extracted and absorbed by the liquid. Teas are infusions. Milk or cream can also be infused with flavor before being used in custards or sauces.

JOINT

To cut meat and poultry into large pieces at the joints using a very sharp knife.

JULIENNE

To cut food into thin sticks. Food is cut with a knife or mandoline into even slices, then into strips.

KNEAD

To mix and work dough into a smooth, elastic mass. Kneading can be done either manually or by machine. By hand, kneading is done with a pressing-folding-turning action. First the dough is pressed with the heels of both hands and pushed away from the body so the dough stretches out. The dough is then folded in half, given a quarter turn, and the process is repeated. Depending on the dough, the kneading time can range anywhere from 5 to 15 minutes. During kneading, the gluten strands stretch and expand, enabling dough to hold in gas bubbles formed by a leavener, which allows it to rise.

LARD

To insert strips of fat (lardons) or bacon into a dry cut of meat using a utensil called a larding needle. Larding makes the cooked meat more succulent and tender.

LINE

To cover the bottom and sides of a cassoulet, mold or terrine with a thin layer of bacon, pork fat, flavorings or pastry. Cake pans are frequently lined with parchment paper to prevent the cake from sticking to the pan after baking.

MACERATE

To soak foods, usually fruit, in liquid so they absorb the liquid's flavor. The macerating liquid is usually alcohol, liqueur, wine, brandy or sugar syrup. Macerate is also frequently applied to fruits sprinkled with sugar, which intensifies natural flavor of the fruit by drawing out its juices.

MARINATE

To soak food in a seasoned liquid mixture for a certain length of time. The purpose of marinating is to add flavor and/or tenderize the food. Due to the acidic ingredients in many marinades, foods should be marinated in glass, ceramic or stainless steel containers. Foods should also be covered and refrigerated while they are marinating. When fruits are soaked in this same manner, the process is called macerating.

MASH

To crush a food into smooth and evenly textured state. For potatoes or other root vegetables, use a ricer, masher or food mill. While food processors provide a smooth texture more like a puree or a paste, they should not be used for potatoes.

MINCE

To cut food into very tiny pieces. Minced food is cut into smaller, finer pieces than diced food.

MOUNT

To whisk cold butter, piece by piece, into a warm sauce for smooth texture, flavor and sheen. Each piece of butter must be thoroughly incorporated before a new piece is added so that the sauce does not break (or separate into liquid and fat).

NAP

To completely coat food with a light, thin, even layer of sauce.

OPEN FACED

A sandwich prepared with just one piece of bread which is topped with a wide variety of meats, vegetables, cheeses and heated or not.

PARBOIL

To boil food briefly in water, cooking it only partially. Parboiling is used for dense food like carrots and potatoes. After being parboiled, these foods can be added at the last minute to quicker-cooking ingredients. Parboiling insures that all ingredients will finish cooking at the same time. Since foods will continue to cook once they have been removed from the boiling water, they should be shocked in ice water briefly to preserve color and texture. Cooking can then be completed by sautéing or the parboiled vegetable can be added to simmering soups or stews.

PARE

To remove the thin outer layer of foods using a paring knife or a vegetable peeler.

PEEL

To remove the rind or skin from a fruit or vegetable using a knife or vegetable peeler.

POACH

To cook food by gently simmering in liquid at or just below the boiling point. The amount of the liquid and poaching temperature depends on the food being poached.

POT ROAST

To cook meat slowly by moist heat in a covered pot. The meat is first browned, then braised either on top of the stove or in the oven. Pot roasting is good for tougher cuts of meat which require longer cooking times to break down connective tissue.

POUND

Pounding thinner cuts of meat tenderizes it by breaking down muscle. Kitchen mallets are generally used for pounding, but it can be done using a small frying pan as well. First place the piece of meat between two pieces of plastic wrap or wax paper.

PUREE

To grind or mash food until completely smooth. This can be done using a food processor or blender or by pressing the food through a sieve.

QUADRILLER

To mark the surface of grilled or broiled food with a crisscross pattern of lines. The scorings are produced by contact with very hot single grill bars which brown the surface of the food. Very hot skewers may also be used to mark the surface.

REDUCE

To thicken or concentrate a liquid by boiling rapidly. The volume of the liquid is reduced as the water evaporates, thereby thickening the consistency and intensifying the flavor.

RICE

To push cooked food through a perforated kitchen tool called a ricer. The resulting food looks like rice.

ROAST

To oven-cook food in an uncovered pan. The food is exposed to high heat which produces a well-browned surface and seals in the juices. Reasonably tender pieces of meat or poultry should be used for roasting. Food that is going to be roasted for a long time may be barded to prevent drying out.

SAUTÉ

To cook food quickly in a small amount of fat or oil, until brown, in a skillet or sauté pan over direct heat. The sauté pan and fat must be hot before the food is added, otherwise the food will absorb oil and become soggy.

SCALD

To dip fruits or vegetables in boiling water in order to loosen their skins and simplify peeling. The produce should be left in the water for only 30 seconds to prohibit cooking, and should be shocked in an ice water bath before the skin is removed.

SCALE

To remove the scales from the skin of a fish using a dull knife or a special kitchen tool called a fish scaler.

SEAR

To brown meat or fish quickly over very high heat either in a fry pan, under a broiler or in a hot oven. Searing seals in the food's juices and provides a crisp tasty exterior. Seared food can then be eaten rare or roasted or braised to desired degree of doneness.

SEASON

To add flavor to foods.

To coat the cooking surface of a new pot or pan with vegetable oil then heat in a 350 degree oven for about an hour. This smoothes out the surface of new pots and pans, particularly cast-iron, and prevents foods from sticking.

SEED

To remove the seeds from fruits and vegetables.

SHRED

To cut food into thin strips. This can be done by hand or by using a grater or food processor. Cooked meat can be shredded by pulling it apart with two forks.

SIEVE

To strain liquids or particles of food through a sieve or strainer. Press the solids, using a ladle or wooden spoon, into the strainer to remove as much liquid and flavor as possible.

SIFT

To pass dry ingredients through a fine mesh sifter so large pieces can be removed. The process also incorporates air to make ingredients like flour, lighter. Synonymous with AERATE.

SIMMER

To cook food in liquid over gentle heat, just below the boiling point, low enough so that tiny bubbles just begin to break the surface.

SKEWER

To spear small pieces of food on long, thin, pointed rods called skewers.

SKIM

To remove the scum that rises to the surface from a liquid when it is boiled. The top layer of the liquid, such as the cream from milk or the foam and fat from stock, soups or sauces, can be removed using a spoon, ladle or skimmer. Soups, stews or sauces can be chilled so that the fat coagulates on the surface and may be easily removed before reheating.

SKIN

To remove the skin from food before or after cooking. Poultry, fish and game are often skinned for reasons of appearance, taste and diet.

SMOKE

To expose fresh food to smoke from a wood fire for a prolonged period of time. Traditionally used for preservation purposes, smoking is now a means of giving flavor to food. Smoking tends to dry the food, kills bacteria, deepens color and gives food a smoky flavor. The duration of smoking varies from 20 minutes to several days. The most commonly used woods are beech, oak and chestnut to which aromatic essences are often added. Small home smokers are now available.

STEAM

To cook food on a rack or in steamer basket over a boiling liquid in a covered pan. Steaming retains flavor, shape, texture, and nutrients better than boiling or poaching.

SUPREME

To remove the flesh sections of citrus fruit from the membranes. Using a sharp knife, cut away all of the skin and pith from the outside of the fruit. Place the knife between the membrane and the flesh of one section and slice down. Turn the knife catching the middle of the fruit. Slice up, removing each section sans membrane.

SWEAT

To cook vegetables in fat over gentle heat so they become soft but not brown, and their juices are concentrated in the cooking fat. If the pan is covered during cooking, the ingredients will keep a certain amount of their natural moisture. If the pan is not covered, the ingredients will remain relatively dry.

TEMPER

1. To slowly bring up the temperature of a cold or room temperature ingredient by adding small amounts of a hot or boiling liquid. Adding the hot liquid gradually prevents the cool ingredient, such as eggs, from cooking or setting. The tempered mixture can then be added back to hot liquid for further cooking. This process is used most in making pastry cream and the like.

2. To bring chocolate to a state in which it has snap, shine and no streaks. Commercially available chocolate is already tempered but this condition changes when it is melted. Tempering is often done when the chocolate will be used for candy making or decorations. Chocolate must be tempered because it contains cocoa butter, a fat that forms crystals after chocolate is melted and cooled. Dull grey streaks form and are called bloom. The classic tempering method is to melt chocolate until it is totally without lumps (semisweet chocolate melts at a temperature of 104 degrees F.) One third of the chocolate is then poured onto a marble slab then spread and

worked back and forth with a metal spatula until it becomes thick and reaches a temperature of about 80 degrees F. The thickened chocolate is then added back to the remaining 2/3 melted chocolate and stirred. The process is repeated until the entire mixture reaches 88-92 degrees for semisweet chocolate, 84-87 degrees for milk or white chocolate.

TENDERIZE

To make meat more tender by pounding with a mallet, marinating for varying periods of time, or storing at lower temperatures. Fat may also be placed into a piece of meat to make it more tender during cooking.

TRUSS

To secure food, usually poultry or game, with string, pins or skewers so that it maintains a compact shape during cooking. Trussing allows for easier basting during cooking.

UNLEAVENED

The word which describes any baked good that has no leavener, such as yeast, baking powder or baking soda.

VANDYKE

To cut zigzags in edges of fruit and vegetables halves, usually oranges, tomatoes or lemons. The food is usually used as a garnish to decorate a dish.

WHIP

To beat ingredients such as egg whites or cream until light and fluffy. Air is incorporated into the ingredients as they are whipped, increasing their volume until they are light and fluffy.

WHISK

To beat ingredients together until smooth, using a kitchen tool called a whisk.

XXX, XXXX, 10X

An indicator on a box of confectioners sugar of how many times it has been ground. The higher the number of X's the finer the grind.

YAKITORI

A Japanese term meaning *"grilled."*

ZEST

To remove the outermost skin layers of citrus fruit using a knife, peeler or zester. When zesting, be careful not to remove the pith, the white layer between the zest and the flesh, which is bitter.

INDEX BY TYPE

ENTREES BREAKFAST

Baked Breakfast 163
Baked Ham and Eggs with Goat
 Cheese 165
Eggs Florentine 169
Italian Style Frittata 166
Baked Eggs 164
Breakfast Skillet 167
Crepes and Fruit 173
Eggs Benedict 171
Waffle 174
Scrambled Eggs and Lox 172
Seafood Omelet 168

BEEF

Basic Low Carb Meatloaf Mixture
 185
Blue Cheese Fillet of Beef 186
Bourbon Steak 198
Braised Beef Short-Ribs 202
Chateaubriand Roast with
 Mushroom Sauce 196
Chimichurri Sauce 71, 193, 194
Classic Veal Osso Buco 188
Easy Home Made Beef Jerky 207
Grilled Herb Steaks 187
Grilled Veal Chop with Morel
 Sauce 206
Horseradish Cream Sauce 200
Open-Faced Steak Sandwich 200
Mexican Flank Steak and Mock
 Tamales 193, 195
Roasted Veal Breast 190
Sauté of Veal Medallions 189
Savory Mushroom-Stuffed Steak
 192

Skillet Tournedos of Beef 201
Southwestern Steak with
 Chipotle Sauce 204
Standing Rib Roast 199
Steak au Poivre 203
Teriyaki Grilled Steak 191
Weekend Barbecued Brisket
 205

LAMB

Braised Lamb Shanks 209
Shepherds Pie 212
Roasted Leg of Lamb
 (Boneless) 211
Roasted Leg of Lamb (Whole)
 210
Simple Grilled or Roasted
 Rack of Lamb 213

MISC.

Flavored mayonnaise 42

PORK

Country Style Ribs and
 Sauerkraut 220
Easy Roast Suckling Pig 224
Italian Style Pork Stir Fry 215
Pork Chops in Low Carb Dill-
 Sour Cream Sauce 216
Pork Chops with Fresh White
 Mushrooms and Tomato
 Chutney 217
Pork Piccata 181, 218
Pork Scaloppini with Creamy
 Caper Sauce 219

RECIPE MAKE OVER

INDEX

T

V

W

ABOUT THE AUTHOR

"I am not a writer; I am a Chef that in 1994 recognized the many benefits of a Low Carb Lifestyle". "My biggest complaint was then and continues to be, the constant attempt by so many to re-create the wheel".

Chef Greg Pryor reveals the simple truths with his new book, "A COMPLETE LOW CARB LIFESTYLE" with the same flair and lay in on the line approach that has shaped his career in the professional culinary field. Professionally trained with a degree in Culinary Arts, this Certified Executive Chef reveals to his readers the knowledge and guidance from many years as a professional Chef, having worked directly with the Atkins Group, applying his training, and creating Low Carb recipes and tips to the Atkins Group. Now Chef Greg shares these and many more recipes and tips to live a Low Carb Lifestyle for Life.